Point-of-care US for Acute Abdomen

Mauro Zago • Marina Troian • Diego Mariani
Editors

Point-of-care US for Acute Abdomen

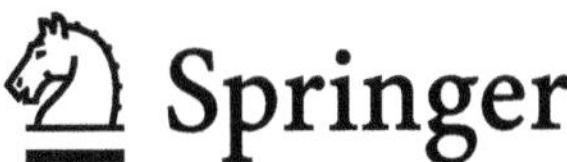

Editors
Mauro Zago
General and Emergency Surgery Unit,
General Surgery Department,
A. Manzoni Hospital
Lecco, Italy

Marina Troian
Cardiothoracic and Vascular Department
ASUGI Cattinara University Hospital
Trieste, Italy

Diego Mariani
ASST OVEST Milanese, General Surgery
Department,
Ospedale di Legnano
Milano, Italy

ISBN 978-3-031-40233-3 ISBN 978-3-031-40231-9 (eBook)
https://doi.org/10.1007/978-3-031-40231-9

This Springer imprint is published by the registered company Springer Nature Switzerland AG
The registered company address is: Gewerbestrasse 11, 6330 Cham, Switzerland

Paper in this product is recyclable.

To our families

To the zamakubi's friendship that never gives up

To the dreamers of MUSEC team

Foreword

The last 30 years have been characterized by an "explosion" of new technology incorporated into daily medical practice. Trauma and emergency general surgery have benefited by the widespread use of imaging modalities applicable to the diagnosis of acute diseases requiring immediate attention and timely intervention, and in the diagnosis of postoperative complications. As technology advanced, the imaging definition became more refined, decreasing interpretation errors and allowing the so-called learning curve to be shorter, thus decreasing the operator dependence, so much debated, particularly in the use of ultrasound.

In fact, ultrasound examinations have become ubiquitous in current surgical practice. Initially performed only by radiologists, the dissemination and accessibility of the method allowed surgeons at all training levels to become quite proficient in the use of ultrasound for the diagnosis of acute abdominal problems, to rule out intraperitoneal and intrapleural blood after trauma, for hemodynamic assessment in the ICU, and as an adjunct to several percutaneous procedures. Ultrasonography is the substitute of the old stethoscope, and in the USA, many first-year medical students receive a portable (pocket) ultrasound instead of a stethoscope.

A decade ago, a group of European acute care surgeons, members of the European Society of Trauma and Emergency Surgery, had the vision to develop a course to train surgeons in the use of this important technology. The Modular UltraSound ESTES Course (MUSEC) has been, continuously in Europe, benefiting a great number of patients with acute surgical problems.

It is with great enthusiasm that I congratulate Drs. Zago, Mariani, and Troian for expanding the initial vision of the MUSEC course and providing us, the learners, with an excellent textbook covering most of the emergency surgery conditions frequently treated by acute care surgeons. Obviously, in some clinical situations, other imaging modalities will be necessary for definitive diagnosis and management. However, its portability, accessibility, and rapid execution make ultrasonography useful as the first and sometimes the only imaging modality used for definitive diagnosis.

The book has 12 chapters written by experts and many instructors of the MUSEC course. It covers most abdominal disease processes, collectively known as "acute abdomen". This book should be a mandatory read for surgical residents, fellows, and junior faculty. In addition, those practicing surgery in low-income countries where ultrasonography is the only (and most sophisticated) imaging modality available will benefit enormously from this publication.

Riverside University Health System
CA USA

Department of Surgery
Loma Linda University School of Medicine
Loma Linda CA USA

Raul Coimbra

Foreword

I am deeply worried about the future of trauma and emergency surgery. The severely injured and critically ill surgical patient is the victim of increasing surgical subspecialization and surgeons who want to restrict their practice to the safety of a limited range of elective procedures.

Trauma is taking more young lives than any other illness. What can be more rewarding than working up, treating, and saving the severely injured and physiologically challenged emergency surgical patients? In order to do so, we need dedication and enthusiasm based on relevant competence, and this again requires quality-assured evidence and training programs for the use of relevant technology.

In the ever-evolving landscape of modern medicine, advancements in technology have played a pivotal role in transforming the field of trauma and emergency surgery. Among the many innovations that have revolutionized patient care, ultrasound has emerged as an indispensable tool, providing clinicians with a rapid, noninvasive, and real-time imaging modality.

This book serves as a comprehensive guide to the benefit and practical use of abdominal ultrasound in emergency surgery, particularly in the setting of the difficult field of the so called acute abdomen. In the face of time-sensitive decisions and the need for accurate diagnoses, ultrasound has become an indispensable asset for healthcare professionals working in trauma and emergency settings. Its versatility lies partly in its ability to rapidly help assess the sick patient, its portability, cost-effectiveness, and safety. The speed at which ultrasound can provide information allows for rapid interventions and optimizing patient care without exposing the patient to unnecessary risks.

However, it is important to keep in mind that the true value is a balance between these benefits and the limitations of this diagnostic tool, defined by clinician experience, competence, and the fact that ultrasound allows the clinician to diagnose, but most often not to exclude a condition.

This book is written by truly dedicated ultrasound specialists and provides the surgical community with a valuable guide to the use of ultrasound. They have harnessed the power of ultrasound to enhance their own practice and elevate the level of care they provide to trauma and emergency surgery patients. Their long-time experience with its clinical application is combined with having run internationally renowned ultrasound training programs for more than a decade, and the book reflects this massive didactic platform.

In conclusion, ultrasound is here to stay! Its benefits and practical use in acute care surgery cannot be overstated provided that it is combined with an understanding of its limitations. This book serves as a comprehensive resource for clinicians seeking to enhance their skills in utilizing ultrasound in critical care settings, and I support the authors when they state that as surgeons, we should all add ultrasound to our diagnostic armamentarium. This book is here to help us!

Oslo University Hospital
Oslo, Norway
Christine Gaarder

Preface

It is with great pleasure that we can offer to the medical and surgical community this practical book, coming from the long-lasting belief and daily experience that ultrasonography (US) can change our attitude in many situations and every time we would like to "see" what is happening *in* our patients.

It is undeniable that US has become a valuable and essential diagnostic and therapeutic tool in everyday clinical practice, easily accessible, portable, and relatively inexpensive. This book is intended to be a practical reference for emergency physicians and surgeons who want to incorporate US diagnostics in the assessment and decision-making process of patients with acute abdominal pain.

We would always like to know what is happening inside the belly of a patient complaining of abdominal pain, wouldn't we? Point-of-care US (POCUS) is the right first step for getting those answers to our questions: sometimes definitely, sometimes partially, and always immediately.

Please hold back the usual refrain: "it is operator-dependent!". Any diagnosis is "operator-dependent" (i.e., it depends on his/her background, skills, experience, etc.), and any medical or surgical gesture needs hard work and dedicated time for learning. But, if you are reading this book, you are still convinced that clinical US is learnable. Allow us to quote Lucas Greiner, fellow and former Secretary of the European Federation of Societies for Ultrasound in Medicine and Biology (EFSUMB): "There is more risk to not do a US than to do it, provided your hand and probe are well connected with your brain."

In this book, we do not aim to provide a comprehensive imaging examination of the gastrointestinal tract, but to answer specific clinical questions with a focused and limited examination. With a design already tested in the previous volume on E-FAST, we try to offer some basic cognitive and visual patterns to apply in the emergency setting for a timely and accurate evaluation of many acute visceral conditions potentially requiring urgent surgical management. Each chapter is centered on the surgical decision-making process, which represents a key point in the diagnostic pathway for both emergency physicians and surgeons.

This book is the product of many collaborators, to all of whom we are deeply indebted for their passionate effort and unlimited dedication. Every work was performed in accordance with current ethical and legal guidelines, and visual resources were taken with permission, using original authors' own materials. This book is also the result of an educational effort that many of the authors contributed to build up, the MUSEC course (Modular UltraSound ESTES Course), which celebrates its tenth anniversary.

Although nothing can replace constant practice, we hope that this textbook will serve as a quick reference guide for both novices and experienced professionals.

Last but not least, we want to extend a special acknowledgment to all the marvelous editorial staff of Springer, especially to Aruna and Donatella, who provided an invaluable support and assistance in preparing this book, maintaining an immense, inexpressible kindness and patience with the editors. We deeply appreciate their efforts.

Lecco, Italy — Mauro Zago
Trieste, Italy — Marina Troian
Milano, Italy — Diego Mariani

Contents

Chapter 1
Why a Surgeon Should Become Proficient in Visceral Point-of-care Ultrasound?

Mauro Zago, Diego Mariani, Jorge Pereira, and Marina Troian

Abdominal pain is a quite common symptom with many potential causes, representing about 4–10% of all emergency department visits. The term *acute abdomen* refers to a sudden, severe abdominal pain that requires urgent and specific care and up to 25% of cases will necessitate surgical treatment.

The patient complaining abdominal pain will usually present with associated signs and symptoms, like fever, nausea, or vomiting. A thorough history and physical examination, as well as adequate evaluation of patient's age and comorbidities, are critical in order to work out a diagnosis. However, almost one third of patients will be diagnosed with non-specific abdominal pain.

Rapid assessment and treatment of acute abdomen are crucial. In this context, a bedside point-of-care ultrasound (POCUS) is the preferred modality for evaluation of the acutely ill patient.

Ultrasonography (US) has been used as a diagnostic imaging tool since the 1950s. At the beginning, the machines were complicated and cumbersome, and dedicated trained personnel was required to acquire and interpret images. Over the

M. Zago
General and Emergency Surgery Unit, General Surgery Department, ASST Lecco, "A. Manzoni" Hospital, Lecco, Italy

D. Mariani
Department of General Surgery, ASST Ovest Milanese, "Ospedale Nuovo" di Legnano, Legnano, Milan, Italy

J. Pereira
Department of General Surgery, Centro Hospitalar Tondela-Viseu, Hospital São Teotónio, Viseu, Portugal

M. Troian (✉)
Cardiothoracic and Vascular Department, Thoracic Surgery Service, ASUGI, Cattinara University Hospital, Trieste, Italy
e-mail: marina.troian@asugi.sanita.fvg.it

M. Zago et al. (eds.), *Point-of-care US for Acute Abdomen*,
https://doi.org/10.1007/978-3-031-40231-9_1

following decades, a significant technological improvement in both equipment and imaging definition determined a widespread application of US to include detailed assessment of almost every organ. Nowadays, US machines have become physically smaller, easily deployable, and more power efficient. The substantial enhancements of transducer sensitivity, imaging processing, and digital technology have resulted in high-quality resolutions and clearer definition. Compared to other medical imaging methods, US has become the ideal diagnostic tool. It is non-invasive, low-cost, and user-friendly. The possibilities of evaluating different clinical scenarios, facilitating accurate bedside examinations, and guiding treatment with the benefit of real-time feedback, have expanded the applications across different specialties. By picking up a US probe, the everyday clinical practice has improved to the extent that any practitioner, either in richest societies or in resource-limited settings, can employ US as a mean to obtain detailed anatomical, physiological, and pathological information as part of the clinical evaluation. Needless to say, the diagnostic power of US comes with an equal potential for diagnostic error, as misdiagnoses, mainly due to inexperience, may worsen patient's condition or determine unnecessary intervention. So, never forget to check the US findings with your clinical reasoning.

1.1 On the Field

Emergency physicians and surgeons, who want to incorporate US in the assessment and decision-making process of patients with acute abdominal pain, deserve admiration, and respect. It would be easier to ask another specialist (in general, a Radiologist) to give you the answers to your clinical suspicions. In the meanwhile, you would be able to take care of other things, but the decision-making process for that patient will probably be delayed. Do you want an example?

Imagine being called to assess a 35-year-old female complaining abdominal pain since the day before. The clinical history and physical examination are suggestive of an acute appendicitis without peritonitis, but considering the age and sex of the patient you cannot exclude an ovulatory colic. Alvarado and AIR scores, providing they can help you, are not available yet as you need lab tests results. Thus, as in use almost everywhere, you will probably ask to run some basic emergency blood samples (if they are not already running) and a US examination (hopefully, not a CT scan) performed by a Radiologist. While waiting for the results, you will be able to get on with your routine, manage other cases, and so on. About an hour will pass before you get back to this patient: it is more or less the time required for getting the lab tests and the Radiologist's report ready to be read. Everything seems quite straightforward, doesn't it?

But let's imagine you can perform POCUS as part of your physical examination, even before labs results. On the one hand, if you find an appendix larger than 6 mm and painful on graded compression, then your suspicion is confirmed and, according to the protocol in use, you can immediately alert the surgeon (if you are not one yourself), you can proceed with the admission of the patient to a surgical ward, you can start setting up the operating room, etc. On the other hand, if you find a moderate amount of fluid, in the absence of signs of peritonitis—even if you cannot visualize the appendix on US—you may think an ovulatory colic is the right diagnosis. You can send her to the Gynecologist… Or, with her permission, you may retrieve a sample of fluid with a US-guided diagnostic peritoneal aspiration (DPA). If the sampled fluid is bloody, then your intuition was right: it is very likely a gynecologic problem.

Do you want another practical example? Imagine you are on a night shift in the surgical ward. You are paged in for a patient on third postoperative day after right hemicolectomy now complaining fever and abdominal pain. On physical examination, the abdomen is tender only in the right quadrants, but vital signs and blood gas analysis are within normal range. You ask to run some emergency blood samples, that will be ready in about 30 minutes. Meanwhile, since the ward is equipped with a US machine, you decide to perform POCUS: you are only capable of performing an E-FAST, but you know your results could prove useful even in the non-trauma setting. And you are right: you find free fluid in all quadrants, too much for saying "it is the remaining fluid after surgery," and considering the abdominal pain complained by the patient, you have all the elements for considering this a postoperative complication. What to do next is up to you.

How many other similar examples can we all remember in our professional lives? We must admit that learning to do and be able to do visceral US are not immediate skills, contrary to FAST and E-FAST. However, like for any POCUS, the aim is not to perform a comprehensive imaging examination of the gastrointestinal tract, but to answer specific clinical questions with a focused and limited examination. Some basic cognitive and visual patterns are enough in the emergency setting for a timely and accurate evaluation of many acute visceral conditions potentially requiring urgent surgical management. Proctored training, constant practice, and the belief that POCUS is really your "sixth sense," can make you more proficient.

1.2 Decision-making

The surgical decision-making process represents a key point in the diagnostic pathway for both emergency physicians and surgeons. The way we build up a decision-making process in our minds is out of the scope of this editorial, as we know it is a complex mix of backgrounds and intuition, the latter not a negligible detail. Some suggested readings at the end of this chapter could be very instructive.

POCUS performed by clinicians in charge of the final decision (i.e., the "owners" of the diagnostic thought process) has much more probability to be guided by intuition: if you cannot find something you were *convinced* of finding, you will either try a little bit harder to find it (i.e., harder than someone who is not involved in the same diagnostic process, like the Radiologist) or you will change your approach and diagnostic hypothesis while performing the US exam. Indeed, you are searching for a *comprehensive* diagnosis, while the Radiologists search for a pathological *image*.

Incorporating US in everyday practice is in the best interest of patients, but it should be equally emphasized that using and understanding US are in the best interest of healthcare providers. Furthermore, POCUS is in the best interest of healthcare systems: shortening time to diagnosis, reducing unnecessary further imaging, anticipating interventional maneuvers, etc., are practical and logical consequences of a systematic use of bedside US, and all entail saving of resources and money, like we will explain in detail in one of the following chapters.

In summary, this book strives to be a source of information in terms of technical details, pitfalls, tips, and tricks, which are derived from the daily clinical and teaching experience of the authors, all of whom are skilled practitioners in this field. Although nothing can replace constant practice, we hope this book will serve as a quick reference guide for both novices and experienced professionals.

Further Reading

Blanco P, Volpicelli G. Common pitfalls in point-of-care ultrasound: a practical guide for emergency and critical care physicians. Crit Ultrasound J. 2016;8(1):15. https://doi.org/10.1186/s13089-016-0052-x.

Latifi R. Surgical decision making. Beyond the evidence based surgery. Springer International Publishing Switzerland; 2016. https://doi.org/10.1007/978-3-319-29824-5.

Law J, Macbeth PB. Ultrasound: from Earth to space. McGill J Med. 2011;13(2):59.

Shiralkar U. Smart surgeons, sharp decisions. Cognitive skills to avoid errors & achieve results. TFM Publishing LTD; 2011.), ISBN: 9781903378816.

Whitson MR, Mayo PH. Ultrasonography in the emergency department. Crit Care. 2016;20(1):227. https://doi.org/10.1186/s13054-016-1399-x.

Chapter 2
US Anatomy of Hollow Viscus

Antonio Rodrigues da Silva, Andrea Casamassima, Julio Constantino, Roser Farré Font, Mercé Güell Farré, and Gary Alan Bass

2.1 Introduction

Ultrasound (US) is a non-invasive, radiation-free, cost-effective, diagnostic method that has been increasingly used in almost every field of medicine. The possibility of evaluating different clinical scenarios, facilitating bedside examination, and guiding treatment makes US a valuable first-line diagnostic tool. The recent technological advancement, as well as the increased experience of physicians, determined a widespread use of US examinations also for the assessment of the gastrointestinal tract,

Supplementary Information The online version contains supplementary material available at https://doi.org/10.1007/978-3-031-40231-9_2.

A. R. da Silva
Department of Surgery, Division of Colorectal Surgery, Hospital Pedro Hispano, Matosinhos, Portugal

A. Casamassima (✉)
Department of General Surgery, ASST Melegnano-Martesana, “Santa Maria delle Stelle” Hospital, Melzo, Milan, Italy

J. Constantino
Department of General Surgery, Centro Hospitalar Tondela-Viseu, Viseu, Portugal

R. Farré Font · M. Güell Farré
Department of General Surgery, Althaia Foundation University Hospital, Manresa, Barcelona, Spain

G. A. Bass
Division of Traumatology, Surgical Critical Care and Emergency Surgery, Penn Presbyterian Medical Center, Philadelphia, USA

M. Zago et al. (eds.), *Point-of-care US for Acute Abdomen*,
https://doi.org/10.1007/978-3-031-40231-9_2

overcoming the supposed difficulty of visualization due to the presence of gas and other intra-luminal contents.

Nowadays, US is considered a safe and reliable imaging method for the diagnosis and follow-up of several diseases like acute appendicitis, acute diverticulitis, inflammatory bowel disease, and small bowel obstruction. However, like in every other US scanning, a good knowledge of both anatomy and physiology is of paramount importance.

2.2 Scanning Technique

It is important to remember that the US image of the bowel very much resembles the normal anatomy. Starting from the outer layer, in the histological sample we recognize the serosa, the longitudinal muscle layer, the circular muscle layer, the submucosa, and the mucosa (Fig. 2.1). In the US image, the same stratification is relatively easy to distinguish, especially when the hollow viscus is filled with fluid.

As you can see in Fig. 2.2, the outermost layer is represented by the serosa, whereas the innermost layer represents the mucosa. The muscular and submucosal layers can be recognized in between.

Under normal circumstances, the stratification of the bowel wall is identified by five stripes of alternating echogenicity. The most inner layer is hyperechogenic and represents the border line between the intestinal lumen and the mucosa, which appears hypoechogenic. Then, the submucosal hyperechogenic layer is identified, followed by the hypoechogenic muscle and the hyperechogenic serous membrane. This stratification is preserved in almost all segments of the gastrointestinal tract, from the stomach down to the left colon, with little variation according to the specific portion (Figs. 2.3, 2.4, 2.5, 2.6, 2.7, 2.8 and 2.9). When the hollow viscus is mostly devoid of contents, or it is filled with feces and/or gas (both hyperechoic), the mucosal membrane is difficult to visualize. Similarly, the serosa is not always

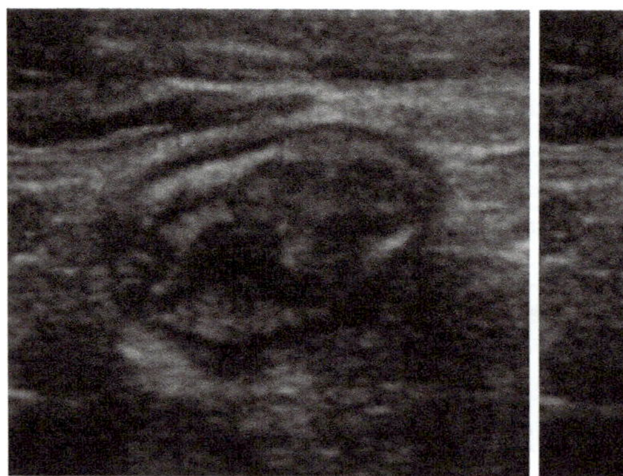
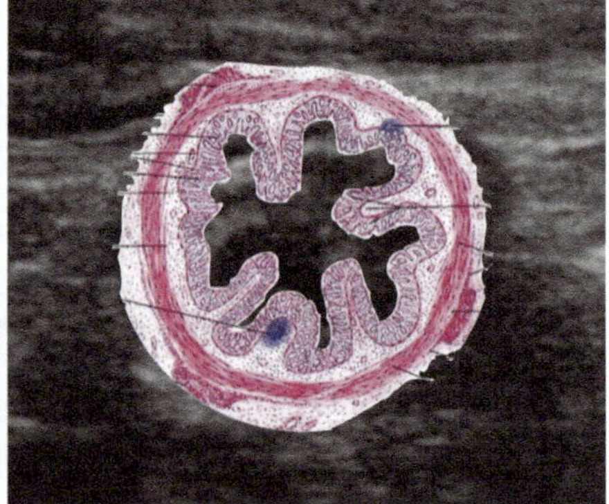

Fig. 2.1 US image (*left*) and reported histological section (*right*) of the bowel wall

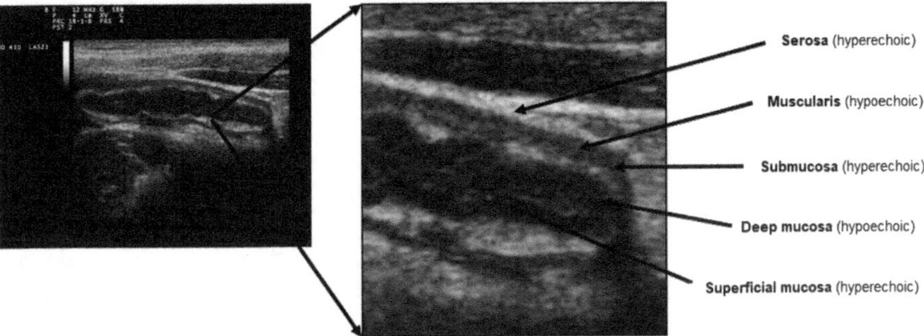

Fig. 2.2 Stratification of the bowel wall (longitudinal axis)

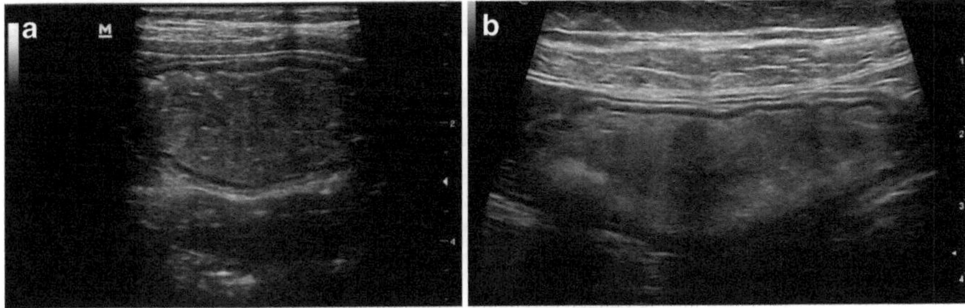

Fig. 2.3 Stomach: very well represented walls, mixed liquid, and gas contents ((**a**): transversal view; (**b**) sagittal view)

clearly visible when adjacent to hyperechoic fat. Thus, most of the times you will be able to see only three layers (i.e., dark deep mucosa—bright submucosa—dark muscularis).

Details on probes and scanning technique are provided in this chapter and in the following chapters for any specific application. In all cases, remember that the linear probe (high frequency) is the preferred probe to be used for visceral US.

In detail, normal anatomy on ultrasound appears as follows:

- **Superficial mucosa**: since it traps little bubbles of gas in between the villi, this layer appears bright white (hyperechoic). However, it is not always visible, especially when adjacent to feces (e.g., in the colon).
- **Deep mucosa**: it appears black (hypoechoic) and it varies in thickness. It contains glands and lymphoid tissue, particularly evident in the last ileal loop of children and young adults (Fig. 2.10).
- **Submucosa**: hyperechoic, it contains the neurovascular fibers of the bowel and loose connective tissue. In patients with inflammatory bowel diseases, vessels are clearly visible when switching from conventional grayscale to Color Flow Doppler mode.
- **Muscularis**: the muscular layer of the bowel wall is easy to identify as it appears as a black circle or stripe (in the axial and longitudinal view, respectively), right below the serosal membrane. It actually consists of two layers, in which fibers

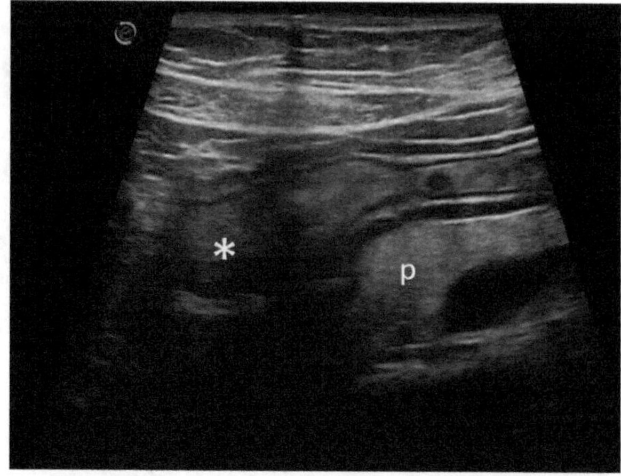

Fig. 2.4 Pylorus, transversal view: very well represented wall (like the stomach), but with a more consistent muscular layer (* pylorus, *p* pancreas)

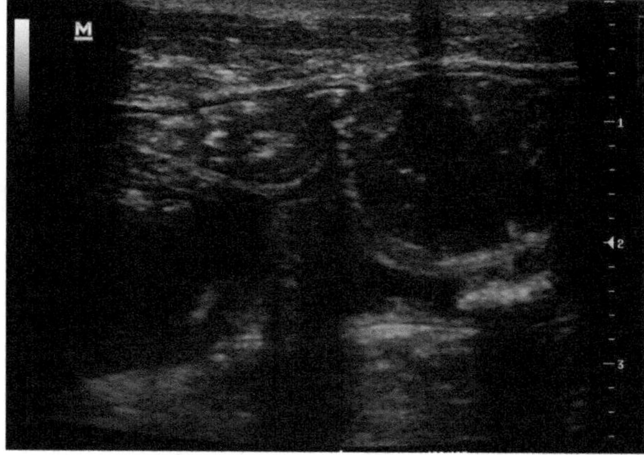

Fig. 2.5 Small bowel: stratification is better visible if the loops are filled with fluid and if there is free fluid in the abdomen between the loops

are stretched in different direction and work cooperatively to produce the peristaltic waves. Sometimes, in lean patients and using a linear probe with very high-resolution power, it is possible to see the thin hyperechoic stripe dividing the circular muscle from the longitudinal muscle. In the large bowel, the teniae could be identified as local thickening of the muscular stratum.

- **Serosa**: it is the outermost hyperechoic layer although not always visible because it is adjacent to the perivisceral fat or omentum (which could appear hyperechoic if inflamed). If there is fluid surrounding the bowel loop, the serosa is clearly visible.

Remember!
- Most of the times you will only see three layers.
- The linear probe is the preferred probe for hollow viscus.

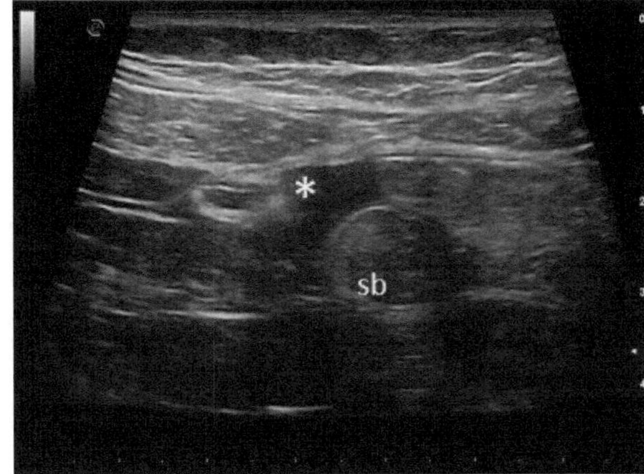

Fig. 2.6 Small bowel: free fluid between the loops (* free fluid, *sb* bowel loop). Free fluid can be recognized due to its pointed contours (not "round shaped")

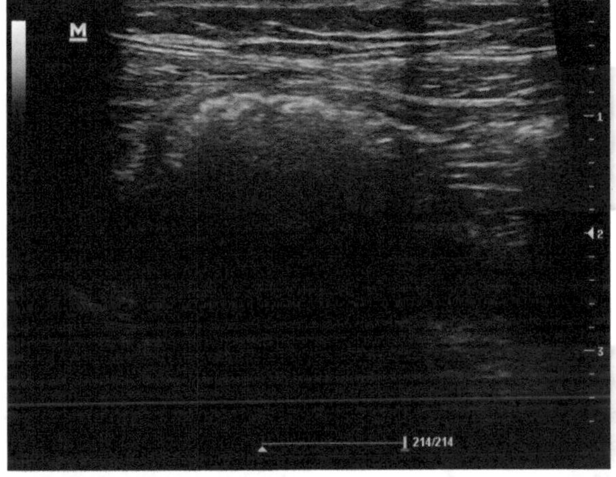

Fig. 2.7 Right colon: not very well visible, thin walls. The posterior wall is hidden by gas artifacts (i.e., white, irregular spots behind the hypoechoic mucosal layer)

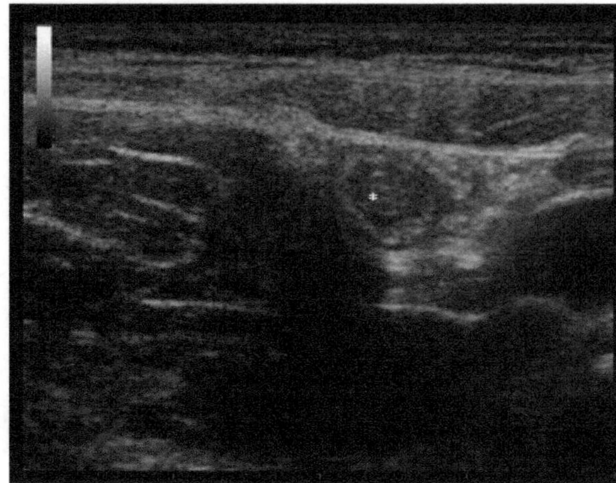

Fig. 2.8 Appendix, transversal view: layered, target-like look (*), not distinguishable from small bowel loop in a single picture! Compressibility and peristalsis (dynamic findings) are absent when looking at the appendix

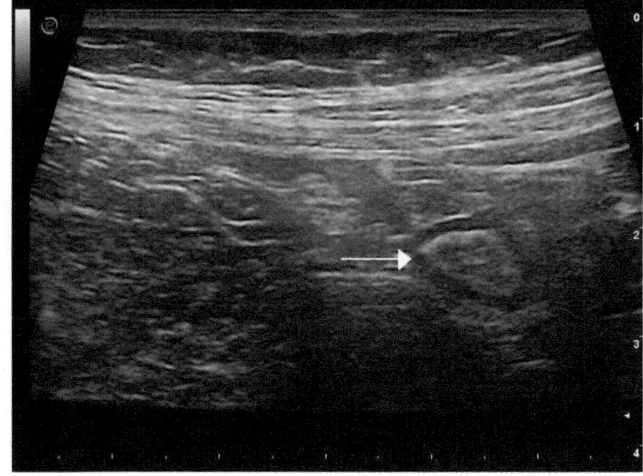

Fig. 2.9 Left colon: compared to the right colon, the left colon presents thicker walls and a smaller diameter (*white arrow*)

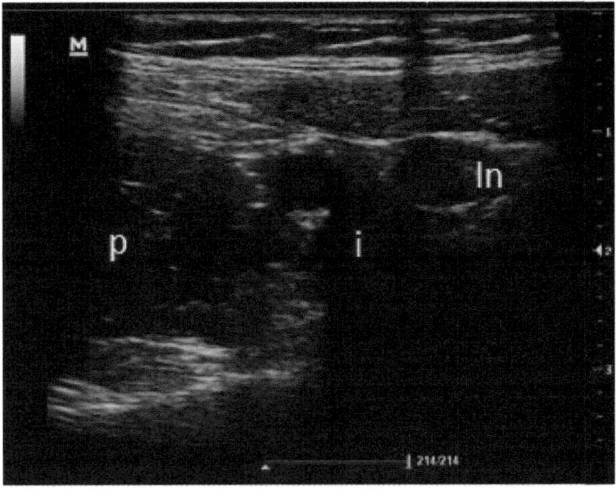

Fig. 2.10 Enlarged lymph nodes in the right lower quadrants can sometimes be found in case of abdominal pain, especially in children and young adults, clinically mimicking an acute appendicitis (*p* psoas, *i* iliac vessels, *ln* lymph node)

Appendix: Chapter 2—Test Yourself (Answers in the Appendix at the End of the Book)

Q1—In the vast majority of cases, how many layers of a hollow viscus can you detect by US?

- 2
- 3
- 4

Q2—Normal peristalsis is easily detectable in the …

- Appendix
- Small bowel
- Large bowel

Further Reading

Pulyaert J. https://radiologyassistant.nl/abdomen/bowel/lk-jg-1-1

Chapter 3
Landmarks and Scanning Technique

Andrea Casamassima, Antonio Rodrigues da Silva, Christos Iordanou, Estela Membrilla, Isidro Martinez Casas, and Marina Troian

3.1 Introduction

The significant technological advancement in both equipment and imaging definition determined a widespread use of ultrasound (US) examination in almost every field of clinical medicine. Being safe, fast, and cheap, US is often the imaging of choice for initial evaluation of the patient presenting with acute abdomen and/or abdominal pain.

Supplementary Information The online version contains supplementary material available at https://doi.org/10.1007/978-3-031-40231-9_3.

A. Casamassima
Department of General Surgery, ASST Melegnano-Martesana, "Santa Maria delle Stelle" Hospital, Melzo, Milan, Italy

A. R. da Silva
Department of Surgery, Division of Colorectal Surgery, Hospital Pedro Hispano, Matosinhos, Portugal

C. Iordanou
Department of Surgery, Thriassio General Hospital, Athens, Greece

E. Membrilla
Division of General and Digestive Surgery, Hospital del Mar, Barcelona, Spain

I. Martinez Casas
Department of General and Digestive Surgery, Virgen del Rocío University Hospital, Seville, Spain

M. Troian (✉)
Cardiothoracic and Vascular Department, Thoracic Surgery Service, ASUGI, Cattinara University Hospital, Trieste, Italy
e-mail: marina.troian@asugi.sanita.fvg.it

M. Zago et al. (eds.), *Point-of-care US for Acute Abdomen*,
https://doi.org/10.1007/978-3-031-40231-9_3

Although the presence of gas and intraluminal contents have historically prevented the application of US to the study of the gastrointestinal tract, the increasing experience acquired by physicians, as well as the technological improvement of machinery, have further increased the application of US in the study of bowel diseases. However, compared to other imaging modalities (e.g., computed tomography, magnetic resonance), intestinal US remains infrequently used in most countries, mostly because of lack of awareness.

3.2 Scanning Technique

The examination of the gastrointestinal tract usually involves the evaluation of the small bowel, colon, and mesentery. Both low-frequency curvilinear probes and high-frequency linear probes are usually required. When performing intestinal US, the bowel wall thickness and layered frame, as well as the motility and vascularity, should be accurately assessed, together with any associated finding regarding adjacent structures (e.g., lymph nodes, fat tissues).

At first, the abdomen is scanned with a low-frequency (3.5–5.0 MHz) convex probe, in order to visualize deeper planes and detect grossly abnormal conditions (e.g., bowel dilation, bowel wall thickening, free fluid, concurrent findings, or alternative diagnoses). Then, you can switch to the high-frequency (5.0–17.0 MHz) linear probe for a more detailed, focused assessment of the presumed pathological condition.

Gradual compression of the bowel wall helps to shift the air within the intestinal lumen, reducing the annoying gas-related artifacts. It could take 2–3 min for getting a clear view of the bowel loops, in the initially "undistinguished grey fog."

Gradual compression also helps to bring the transducer closer to the bowel, providing a better view. Under normal circumstances, healthy bowel and adjacent soft tissues are easy to compress. Any stiffness during continuous, gradual compression should be regarded as abnormal.

Gradual compression could also elicit pain. Evaluating the painful underlying structure can give you immediate and precise clinical information. For instance, a painful uncompressible appendix under the probe is quite pathognomonic, but pain elicited over a normal bowel loop, or the psoas muscle, redirects you to an alternative diagnosis.

Preset. The choice of a proper preset is particularly important in the visceral US. Most modern equipment have a specific "intestinal" preset, applied to the linear probe. If in doubt, ask the specialist to help you arrange one.

If your US equipment does not (yet) have a dedicated preset for visceral examination, check the best one among those available. Suggestions: thyroid or testicle preset could be ok, but deep view will be lost very soon; small part preset is usually inappropriate; pediatric abdomen or generic abdomen presets are sometimes the only acceptable compromise.

3.3 Location and Landmarks

When performing intestinal US, it appears useful to start the assessment at an area with a known fixed location. Specifically, the large bowel frames the abdomen, with the right and left colon being fixed in the paracolic gutters. The cecum, transverse colon, and sigmoid colon can move and be longer than expected.

The small bowel is generally more variable in position although in most patients the jejunum can be found in the upper left quadrants and the ileum in the right lower quadrants. In this context, an important landmark is represented by the terminal ileum, located close to the ileocecal valve. In other words, do not forget normal real anatomy when performing intestinal US.

If you are a beginner in this field, you could be fully absorbed by the US screen. If you get lost, step back to the normal anatomy and restart POCUS.

Luminal appearance. The small bowel typically presents a smaller diameter, with fluid contents and mucosal folds (i.e., valvulae conniventes), which are generally more evident in the jejunum rather than in the ileum. Conversely, the colon has a larger caliber and is usually filled with gas and feces determining its hyperechoic appearance with slight US beam attenuation.

Another feature characterizing the small bowel is the presence of peristalsis, which is normally not seen in the colon due to its slower movements.

Bowel wall stratification. Conventional grey-scale US allows the identification of all five layers of the intestinal wall, resulting from a combination of interface echoes determining different grades of echogenicity. The inner layer is hyperechoic and is determined by the interface between the mucosa and the lumen. Then, there is a hypoechoic stripe, corresponding to the deep mucosa, followed by another hyperechoic stripe, representing the submucosal membrane, and one more hypoechoic layer, composing the muscular fibers. The outer hyperechoic layer corresponds to the serosa.

When the bowel is devoid of contents, or when it is filled with feces, the mucosa can be difficult to visualize as gas and feces are both hyperechoic. Similarly, the serosal layer is generally very thin and not always visible. Therefore, most of the times you will detect only three alternating layers (i.e., black mucosa—white submucosa–black muscularis).

Another important parameter to register when performing intestinal US is bowel wall thickness. In normal individuals, the intestinal wall measures up to 3–4 mm in the small bowel and up to 4 mm in the colon. Increased thickness is generally associated with pathologic conditions, such as inflammation and cancer.

Bowel wall vascularization. Intestinal US examination can be enhanced by Doppler mode and Color Flow mapping, which can provide additional information on the status of bowel wall vascularization, based on the intensity of color signals and Doppler curves.

Healthy bowel is generally without significant color Doppler signal. On the contrary, an increased and hyperdynamic flow will be recorded in case of acute inflammation. A proper setting of the velocity flow assessment and the ability of the patient to hold the breath is mandatory for getting reliable images.

However, it should be noted that Doppler imaging techniques allow only the detection of large vessels and may not provide adequate information on the microcirculation. Power Doppler can increase the sensitivity for the detection of low velocity flow. In this context, the performance can be further enhanced using high-frequency linear probes after intravenous administration of contrast media (CEUS—Contrast-Enhanced UltraSound) (see Chap. 9).

Assessment of adjacent structures. A complete intestinal US cannot elude an accurate assessment of the adjacent mesentery, omentum, and lymph nodes. For example, in case of acute inflammation, the perivisceral fat tissue will appear non-compressible, relatively hyperechoic (the equivalent of the "fat stranding" on CT) and with increased vascularity. Free fluid may be present between the loops and could be retrieved and analyzed by a US-guided Diagnostic Peritoneal Aspiration (DPA).

Lymph nodes are common findings during US assessment of the gastrointestinal tract. However, enlarged lymph nodes (diameter >10 mm) could be associated with inflammatory, infectious, and neoplastic processes. Sometimes, in children and young adults, they may be responsible for abdominal pain (i.e., mesenteric lymphadenitis), mimicking acute appendicitis.

Remember!

- Convex probe first, linear probe after.
- Always check for the best preset.
- Be patient! Wait a few minutes and the "grey fog" will lift.
- Gentle graded compression is of paramount importance: it allows you to get the target, assess compressibility, and evaluate focused pain.
- Measure thickness of the bowel wall.
- Enhance your exam with DPA if free fluid is found and its nature is relevant for the clinical decision-making process.

Chapter 4
Bowel Obstruction: The Clinical Questions Can Be Answered by US

Matteo Marconi, Hayato Kurihara, Isidro Martinez Casas, Erol Erden Ünlüer, Jacopo Guerrini, and Mauro Zago

4.1 Introduction

Small bowel obstruction (SBO) is a relatively common presentation to the Emergency Department (ED), accounting for up to 15% of surgical admissions. It is determined by a variety of pathologic processes leading to an either partial or complete obstruction of the normal intestinal transit. In industrialized countries, the main cause of SBO is postoperative adhesions (65–75%), followed by hernias,

Supplementary Information The online version contains supplementary material available at https://doi.org/10.1007/978-3-031-40231-9_4.

M. Marconi (✉)
General Surgery Department, ASST Ovest Milanese, "G. Fornaroli" Hospital, Magenta, Milan, Italy

H. Kurihara
Department of Emergency Surgery, Fondazione IRCCS Ca' Granda, Ospedale Maggiore Policlinico, Milan, Italy

I. Martinez Casas
Department of General and Digestive Surgery, Virgen del Rocío University Hospital, Seville, Spain

E. E. Ünlüer
Emergency Medicine Department, University of Health Sciences İzmir Bozyaka Education and Research Hospital, İzmir, Turkey

J. Guerrini
Department of General Surgery, ASL TO5, Ospedale Maggiore, Chieri, Turin, Italy

M. Zago
General and Emergency Surgery Unit, General Surgery Department, ASST Lecco, "A. Manzoni" Hospital, Lecco, Italy

M. Zago et al. (eds.), *Point-of-care US for Acute Abdomen*,
https://doi.org/10.1007/978-3-031-40231-9_4

malignancy, and inflammatory diseases (e.g., Crohn disease). The management of bowel obstruction depends on the etiology, severity, and location of the obstruction, but most cases do not require operative intervention and SBO can be managed conservatively with gastric tube insertion, bowel rest, and intravenous fluids. Multimodality imaging has been proposed to confirm, stage, and define the cause of SBO. Abdominal plain film radiography is often the initial study, but with an overall sensitivity of less than 70% it is frequently non-diagnostic, and it should be abandoned. Contrast-enhanced computed tomography (CT) represents the gold-standard imaging modality in the evaluation of SBO, answering to all diagnostic key points. In fact, it can confirm the pathology, determine the cause and level of mechanical obstruction, and stage SBO, defining the presence or absence of parietal damage. However, CT imaging is time-consuming, expensive, not always readily available, and it exposes the patient to ionizing radiation. Recent studies demonstrated that ultrasound (US) and bedside point-of-care ultrasound (POCUS) have a reasonably high accuracy in diagnosing SBO compared with CT scan, representing a rapid diagnostic modality to determine the presence or absence of pathology and substantially decreasing the time to diagnosis. It is easy to use and highly accessible, it can be performed bedside, and it requires no radiation exposure, thus potentially decreasing healthcare costs.

4.2 Scanning Technique

Ultrasound examination of the small bowel is usually performed with the patient in a supine position. A 3.5–5.0 MHz curvilinear probe at an imaging depth of 12–18 cm according with the size of the patient is used to obtain a general overview of the abdomen. A 7.0–12.0 MHz linear transducer may be used for a thin patient and always for better assessment of more superficial loops and the presence of free fluids in between bowel loops.

The small bowel is located in the central regions of the abdomen and should be searched in a systematic fashion to ensure that no area is left unscanned. Begin the scanning in one of the paracolic gutters and sweep along the course of the flank on each side, or from the epigastrium down to the pelvis, in a method described as "*mowing-the-lawn*" technique (Fig. 4.1).

Compression should be graded and gentle, in order not to cause pain and to avoid pushing the bowel out of the US plane. Interference by gas echoes from distended bowel can be avoided by scanning the distended abdomen using oblique or coronal planes, or by applying gentle pressure when moving the transducer slowly over the abdomen with the purpose of squeezing the air away from the region of interest. The linear probe can then be used for focused examination of referred points of focal tenderness.

General limitations to performing POCUS for SBO include significant amount of bowel gas, obesity, patient positioning, and operator experience. Normal small bowel is easily recognized on US by its characteristic mural stratification, with

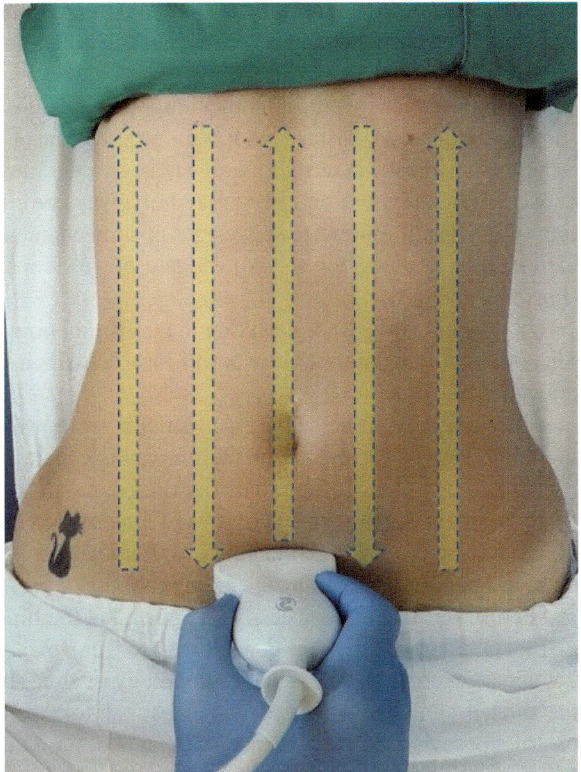

Fig. 4.1 "Mowing-the-lawn" technique

alternating circles of contrasting echogenicity, and its continuous and vivid peristalsis, even if the lumen is empty.

Normal anatomy and basic abnormal findings. The jejunum is mainly located in the left upper quadrant and contains more mucosal folds (i.e., valvulae conniventes or Kerckring's folds) than the ileum, which is usually located more in the right lower quadrant and presents with sparse or absent mucosal folds. The terminal ileum can often be separately identified due to its specific location, and it is frequently followed until it disappears into the feces-filled cecum.

The layered wall structure and thickness of the small bowel may change with disease. Usually, the normal small bowel is compressible, and it presents five sonographic layers that result from a combination of interface echoes and the US characteristics of the different histological layers. The most inner hyperechoic layer is defined by the interface between the mucosa and the lumen and is followed by a hypoechoic layer which corresponds to the actual mucosa. The middle hyperechoic layer represents the submucosa and precedes another hypoechoic layer corresponding to most of the proper muscle. The outer hyperechoic layer corresponds to the interface between the proper muscle and the serosa. Since the thin hyperechoic interface from the serosa is variably visible, the overall wall thickness should be measured under mild compression from just above the air-mucosal interface to the outside of the proper muscle layer border. Although measuring wall thickness can be difficult because it changes with peristalsis, small bowel wall in the normal individual is less than 3 mm.

The bowel movement is another important feature to assess. Early SBO may show an increased peristalsis, but with progression of the obstruction, bowel wall ischemia may ensue determining reduced or absent movements. The differentiation between dynamic ileus and SBO may not always be simple. Ideally, the visualization of a transition point is suggestive of a mechanical obstruction, and it can be identified by looking for areas of dilated bowel loops adjacent to collapsed ones (Figs. 4.2 and 4.3).

US is rarely enough for detecting the transition point, but its sensitivity for identification of dilated/non-dilated bowel loops entails a very high sensitivity for the diagnosis of SBO.

Other findings, more suggestive of ileus, are bowel filled with gas, rather than fluid, and lack of peristalsis. In addition, an adequate and complete patient history is also critical to help differentiate between dynamic and mechanical conditions.

Assessment of peristaltic activity and lumen compressibility are two advantages of US over other imaging modalities. Wall thickening, disrupting of the characteristic mural pattern, and derangement of peristaltic waves are common to many small bowel diseases and may be easily recognized at the time of POCUS.

Extent of obstruction is generally based on involvement of the stomach and colonic segments, as well as the morphology of small bowel loops. The location of the dilated small bowel loops and intestinal fold pattern determine the level of obstruction, whereas the presence of other abdominal findings may help in the differential diagnosis (e.g., the presence of liver metastases may suggest a neoplastic obstruction; portal venous gas, manifesting as echogenic mobile foci in the lumen of the portal vein, may be indicative of ischemic bowel disease).

Even though the specific criteria for US diagnosis of SBO varies in medical literature, most publications agree on the main findings, as reported in Table 4.1.

In the last decades, improvements in US technology and wide application of POCUS in the ED has led to an increasing use of this imaging modality in the

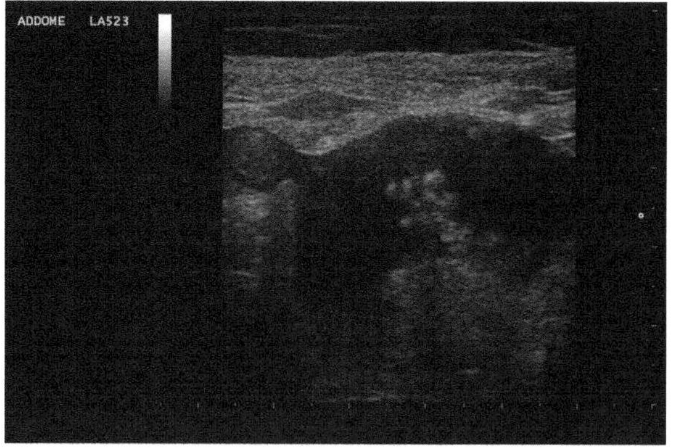

Fig. 4.2 Dilated bowel loop adjacent to a normal one

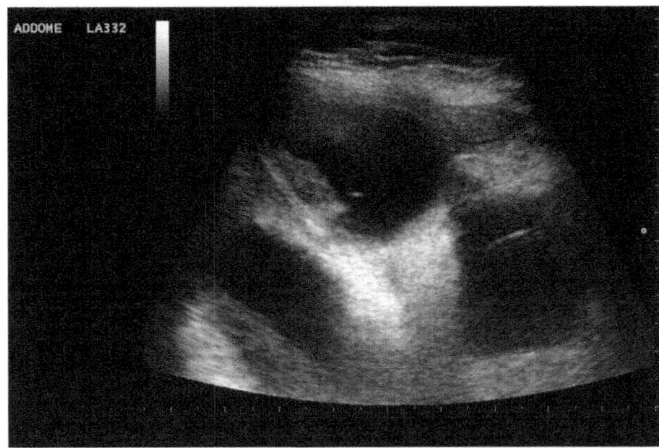

Fig. 4.3 Ileum with thickened walls, filled with air, stools and liquid, adjacent to a normal loop

Table 4.1 US findings of SBO

- Presence of fluid-filled, **dilated bowel loops** (Ø ≥ 25 mm), proximal to normal or collapsed bowel.
- Absent or **ineffective peristalsis**, resulting in back-and-forth movements of spot echoes inside the fluid-filled loops (also referred to as "to-and-fro" or "whirling" appearance of intra-luminal contents).
- **Free fluid** between the dilated loops (the "pointy" triangular appearance of inter-loop free fluid is often referred to as the "tanga sign").
- **Collapsed colonic lumen**.

assessment of patients with possible SBO, as it can be performed quickly, at the patient's bedside, and with no associated radiation exposure. According to literature data, when performed by radiologists, US has a sensitivity of 95% and a specificity of 84% for SBO, whereas the reported sensitivity of plain film radiography is 59–77%.

In 2010, Ünlüer and colleagues prospectively evaluated the diagnostic accuracy of POCUS in the assessment of 174 patients presenting to the ED with suspected SBO. In their study, emergency medicine residents performed US after a 6-h training program. The exam was deemed positive when at least two of the following US features were found: dilated small bowel loops in three segments, increased peristalsis, and collapsed colonic lumen. Results were compared with surgical findings when patients were operated, or self-reported condition at 1-month follow-up. The authors described an overall sensitivity and specificity of 97.7% and 92.7%, respectively, with dilated bowel loops having the best diagnostic accuracy (sensitivity 94.2%, specificity 93.8%). Similarly, in 2011, Jang and colleagues prospectively evaluated the diagnostic accuracy of US performed by trained emergency medicine residents on 76 patients with suspected SBO. A positive US was defined by the presence of at least one of the following criteria: fluid-filled, dilated bowel loops (>25 mm) proximal to collapsed or normal bowel, and/or decreased peristalsis. Results were compared to CT scan images and the authors reported a sensitivity of 93.9% and a specificity of 81.4%.

The results of these studies were further confirmed in 2017 by Gottlieb and colleagues, who published a systematic review and meta-analysis of the use of US to evaluate SBO. According to their analysis, including 11 studies with 1178 patients, US performed by ED physicians, surgeons, and radiologists was found to be 92.4% sensitive and 96.6% specific for SBO. Hence, considering all data so far, POCUS for SBO is easily learned, can be accurately performed by ED physicians and surgeons, and has the potential to expedite surgical consultation and treatment prior to obtaining a CT scan, skipping the use of plain abdominal X-rays.

4.3 Clinical Meanings of Abnormal Findings

As for any POCUS, clinical questions are of paramount importance. When scanning the abdomen for possible SBO (your *main* clinical issue!), what questions should be answered by US? We reported a scheme in Table 4.2.

Because SBO is a dynamic pathology that can either resolve or evolve, accurate staging of SBO is extremely important. From a pathophysiological point of view, the mechanical obstacle to the normal intestinal transit initially determines bowel dilation and fluid-filled loops. The bowels proximal to the point of obstruction may present increased peristaltic movements, trying to overcome the obstacle, and the mucosal folds may be clearly visible although not yet thickened. With the persistence of the mechanical obstruction, the movements will progressively decrease, while the increasing endoluminal pressure will determine an impairment in bowel's ability to re-absorb liquids, thus allowing the passage of fluid in the peritoneal cavity. On US imaging, one of the first signs indicating a worsening of the condition is the presence of extraluminal-free fluid between the bowel loops. The bowel will appear dilated, with thickened mucosal folds ("keyboard sign") and rare or absent movements (Fig. 4.4). As time passes, vascular damage will progress involving the whole bowel wall, which will appear thickened and with parietal stratification on US. Some US findings are suggestive of bowel ischemia and/or infarction and prompt urgent surgical evaluation (Table 4.3).

The presence of free fluid between the bowel loops and in the abdominal recesses is particularly suggestive of worsening mechanical SBO, requiring immediate surgical attention. The key question now is the following: *which is the color/nature of the free fluid*?

Table 4.2 Key questions when performing POCUS for SBO

- Is the small bowel fluid-filled?
- Is the small bowel dilated (i.e., ≥25 mm in outer diameter)?
- Is the small bowel wall thickened (≥3 mm)?
- Is there a distal collapsed segment? Is there a transition point visible?
- It there any peristaltic movement within the small bowel wall? If yes, is it effective?
- Is there free fluid between the small bowel loops?

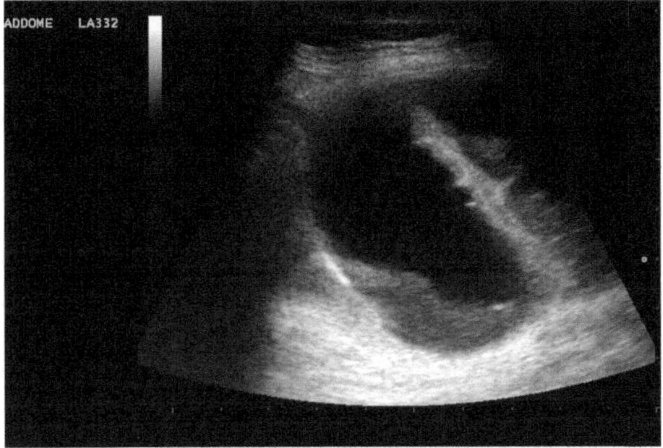

Fig. 4.4 Long lasting occlusion with loss of bowel loops normal anatomy

Table 4.3 US findings suggestive of bowel ischemia and/or infarction

- **Extraluminal free fluid**
  - It is initially anechoic, containing no floating particles or fibrin strands (transudate).
  - With the worsening of mechanical SBO, inflammation and infection of the peritoneum determines the presence of an exudate, containing echogenic filamentous septa and adhesions.
- **Loss of peristalsis**
- **Bowel wall thickening > 3 mm, with disrupted mural architecture.**
- **Mural gas**

As US can detect as little as 100 mL of fluid, a US-guided diagnostic peritoneal aspiration (DPA) can be performed for diagnostic evaluation of the fluid (i.e., serum, blood, bile, pus, enteric contents). In this case, by means of a low frequency transducer (3.5 MHz), the easiest detectable pocket of fluid is identified, with the most suitable probe (convex or linear), and an 18–21 Gauge needle is inserted through the abdominal wall under real-time US guidance. The tip of the needle appears as a hyperechoic pointed structure and care should be taken to steer clear of the moving bowel and the bladder. The quality of the fluid can help the decision-making process of the patient's management.

Among the many causes of SBO, small bowel invagination is one of the most common causes of acute abdomen in children, especially within the early years of age. It occurs when a proximal bowel loop is pulled forward into itself, and it determines an obstruction which may potentially evolve into mesenteric vascular compromise and bowel ischemia, if not promptly recognized. In small children, a lead point is usually not identified, and the cause of intussusception is thought to be related to the presence of hypertrophic lymphoid tissue, maybe following a gastrointestinal infection. On the contrary, in adults it is usually caused by a focal lesion acting as a lead point (e.g., benign or malignant neoplasms, congenital duplication cyst, Meckel diverticulum). US has a sensitivity of nearly 100% and a specificity of about 90% in experienced hands, so that a negative study can generally rule out intussusception. The most characteristic sign of intussusception on US is the "target sign" (also known as "onion sign," "doughnut sign," "bull's eye sign," or "coiled spring sign"), which is generated by concentric alternating echogenic and hypoechoic bands represented by the layers of the invaginated intestine when seen in the transversal plane. When the mesentery is involved, this forms a hyperechoic crescent open towards the antimesenteric side ("crescent in the doughnut sign"). When seen longitudinally, the mesentery is seen as a hyperechoic layer between two multilayered structures (the "sandwich sign"). Intussusception can occur essentially anywhere, although the most common site is ileocolic, probably due to the abundance of lymphoid tissue in the terminal ileum and the anatomy of the ileocecal region. Therefore, the "target sign" will usually be apparent in the right lower quadrant. Color Doppler imaging may reveal a lack of perfusion in the wall of the invaginated bowel, indicating the potential development of ischemia and warranting immediate surgical attention.

Tips and Tricks

- Compression should be graded and gentle.
  - Do not cause pain.
  - Once the air has been displaced, slide the probe while continuing to compress to prevent re-accumulation of gas in the visualized segment.
- Examine the abdomen in a systematic fashion to ensure that a dilated and distended segment is not missed.
  - On initial assessment, it is reasonable to begin at the maximal point of tenderness, where it is more likely for a mechanical obstruction to be identified.
- A curvilinear probe provides the best penetration and image resolution for identifying SBO in most patients.
  - In selected cases, with minimal adipose tissue, a linear probe can be acceptable, but remember that the depth of visualization will be limited.

Remember!

- **Be patient!** Many of the earliest findings of an SBO (e.g., "to-and-fro" movements or lack of peristalsis) will be identified only when the bowel is viewed repeatedly over time.
- **Warning**: if an obstruction is identified, continue the examination of the bowel until it can be deemed to be complete, so you don't miss other potential causes of obstruction (e.g., hernias, intussusceptions, abscesses, and masses).
- **Warning**: know your limitation! POCUS can identify SBO but will not rule it out and might not identify the cause. The concern for ischemic bowel must remain high.
- **Enhance your exam with DPA**, if free fluid is found and its actual nature is clinically relevant.

Appendix: Chapter 4—Test Yourself (Answers in the Appendix at the End of the Book)

Q1—Look at Fig. 4. How dilated is the bowel loop?

- 20 mm
- 30 mm
- 50 mm

Q2—What do you need to search for confirming an SBO on US?

- dilated stomach
- dilated colon
- empty distal small bowel

Further Reading

Atkinson NSS, Bryant RV, Dong Y, Maaser C, Kucharzik T, Maconi G, et al. How to perform gastrointestinal ultrasound: Anatomy and normal findings. World J Gastroenterol. 2017;23(38):6931–41. https://doi.org/10.3748/wjg.v23.i38.6931.

Frasure SE, Hildreth AF, Seethala R, Kimberly HH. Accuracy of abdominal ultrasound for the diagnosis of small bowel obstruction in the emergency department. World J Emerg Med. 2018;9(4):267–71. https://doi.org/10.5847/wjem.j.1920-8642.2018.04.005.

Gottlieb M, Peksa GD, Pandurangadu AV, Nakitende D, Takhar S, Seethala RR. Utilization of ultrasound for the evaluation of small bowel obstruction: a systematic review and meta-analysis. Am J Emerg Med. 2018;36(2):234–42. https://doi.org/10.1016/j.ajem.2017.07.085.

Guttman J, Stone MB, Kimberly HH, Rempell JS. Point-of-care ultrasonography for the diagnosis of small bowel obstruction in the emergency department. CJEM. 2015;17(2):206–9. https://doi.org/10.2310/8000.2014.141382.

Jang TB, Schindler D, Kaji AH. Bedside ultrasonography for the detection of small bowel obstruction in the emergency department. Emerg Med J. 2011;28(8):676–8. https://doi.org/10.1136/emj.2010.09572.

Nylund K, Ødegaard S, Hausken T, Folvik G, Lied GA, Viola I, et al. Sonography of the small intestine. World J Gastroenterol. 2009;15(11):1319–30. https://doi.org/10.3748/wjg.15.1319.

Pourmand A, Dimbil U, Drake A, Shokoohi H. The accuracy of point-of-care ultrasound in detecting small bowel obstruction in emergency department. Emerg Med Int. 2018;(2018):3684081. https://doi.org/10.1155/2018/3684081.

Unlüer EE, Yavaşi O, Eroğlu O, Yilmaz C, Akarca FK. Ultrasonography by emergency medicine and radiology residents for the diagnosis of small bowel obstruction. Eur J Emerg Med. 2010;17(5):260–4. https://doi.org/10.1097/MEJ.0b013e328336c736.

Chapter 5
Acute Diverticulitis: US Diagnosis and Staging

Mauro Zago, Daniel Bogdan Dumbrava, Diego Mariani, Gary Alan Bass, Luca Ponchietti, and Alan Biloslavo

5.1 Introduction

Acute diverticulitis is one of the commonest conditions dealt with in surgical practice, as well as one of the most frequent abdominal emergencies managed non-operatively. It is the second leading cause of abdominal pain in adults and represents a significant burden on healthcare services throughout the world in terms of hospital admissions, outpatient visits, and diagnostic procedures.

Supplementary Information The online version contains supplementary material available at https://doi.org/10.1007/978-3-031-40231-9_5.

M. Zago (✉)
General and Emergency Surgery Unit, General Surgery Department, ASST Lecco, "A. Manzoni" Hospital, Lecco, Italy

D. B. Dumbrava
General Surgery Department, Ponderas Academic Hospital, Bucharest, Romania

D. Mariani
Department of General Surgery, ASST Ovest Milanese, "Ospedale Nuovo" di Legnano, Legnano, Milan, Italy

G. A. Bass
Division of Traumatology, Surgical Critical Care and Emergency Surgery, Penn Presbyterian Medical Center, Philadelphia, PA, USA

L. Ponchietti
Department of General Surgery, San Jorge Hospital, Huesca, Spain

A. Biloslavo
Department of General Surgery, ASUGI, Cattinara University Hospital, Trieste, Italy

M. Zago et al. (eds.), *Point-of-care US for Acute Abdomen*,
https://doi.org/10.1007/978-3-031-40231-9_5

Diverticular disease is characterized by outpouchings of the colonic layers and is determined by multiple factors, including slow bowel transit, high intraluminal pressure, and weakened colonic wall. The sigmoid colon is involved in more than 90% of cases and diverticula can usually occur adjacent to the vasa recta, on the mesenteric side of the colon. Acute inflammation stems from obstruction of the thin-walled diverticulum by a fecalith, which causes stagnation and bacterial overgrowth activating an inflammatory response. Although most patients presenting with acute inflammation will have an indolent course and will be discharged without surgical intervention, up to 10–20% of patients will develop complications and may require emergency surgery. Moreover, it must be noted that still a high proportion of non-complicated acute diverticulitis are admitted to hospital wards although they could be treated in an outpatient setting.

Although challenging, the diagnosis and classification of severity of acute diverticulitis are of paramount importance. A thorough history and clinical examination are essential, but not every patient will present with the classical picture of left lower quadrant pain, fever, and leukocytosis. In addition, the rate of misdiagnosis can be quite high as not every patient presenting with these symptoms suffers from acute diverticulitis. In this context, contrast-enhanced computed tomography (CT) of the abdomen and pelvis is currently the standard imaging technique in suspected acute colonic diverticulitis, allowing for accurate evaluation and staging of colonic inflammation as well as planning of possible percutaneous interventions. Based on clinical and radiological findings, patients can be categorized in different grades of increasing severity. Notwithstanding ongoing proposals, the simplicity of the grading system still makes the modified Hinchey classification the most used classification tool, dividing patients into four grades of increasing clinical severity (Table 5.1).

CT scanning has a reported sensitivity of 93% for the diagnosis of acute diverticulitis. However, false-negative results can occur in the early stage of disease, as the pericolic fat may have only minor changes. Similarly, false-positive results can happen as increased attenuation in the pericolic fat is not specific for diverticulitis and differential diagnosis includes colon cancer, inflammatory bowel disease, and acute inflammation of epiploic appendages. In addition, CT scanning carries other

Table 5.1 Modified Hinchey classification (adapted from *Wasvary et al., Am Surg 1999; 65(7):632-5*).

Score	Modified Hinchey classification	CT findings
0	Mild clinical diverticulitis	Thickened colonic wall, diverticula
1A	Confined pericolic inflammation / phlegmon	Thickened colonic wall, soft tissue changes
1B	Confined pericolic abscess	Thickened colonic wall, soft tissue changes, localized abscess
2	Pelvic or distant abscess	Thickened colonic wall, soft tissue changes, distant abscess
3	Purulent peritonitis	Free intraperitoneal gas and fluid
4	Fecal peritonitis	Free intraperitoneal gas and fluid suggestive for fecal matter

restrictions, like the potential limited availability after-hours, higher costs, the need for contrast media, and radiation exposure.

In acute diverticulitis, ultrasound (US) is particularly attractive because it allows definition of the extent of extra-mucosal inflammatory masses as well as the identification of abscesses, with a reported sensitivity of 85% and specificity of 84%, respectively. US has been recently included in imaging algorithms and society guidelines as a primary diagnostic tool, especially in the emergency department. Recent papers have demonstrated that US can get an accuracy comparable to CT in grading the severity of the disease, in particular for low-grade Hinchey scores, allowing for a simplified path in the outpatient management of non-complicated acute diverticulitis patients. Complementary to clinical evaluation, CT scanning, and colonoscopy, US allows to "fill the gap" between the low accuracy of simple physical examination and the high costs and related risks of a CT scan.

5.2 Scanning Technique

Because of its lateral location in the left paracolic gutter, the normal descending and sigmoid colon can be easily identified in almost every patient. The normal appearance will be variable, depending on whether the lumen is empty or filled with feces. Both convex (2.5–5.0 MHz) and linear (5.0–12.0) probes are used for evaluation: the higher the frequency, the better the assessment of the large bowel in non-obese patients. Conversely, the convex, low-frequency probe could be the only one useful in scanning obese patients.

Use first the low-frequency probe, for an overall evaluation of the abdomen and gross scanning of the target area, looking for intraperitoneal-free fluid and/or pathological findings of adjacent structures. Then, change to the linear high-frequency probe to obtain more detailed images of the normal anatomy and changes in the bowel wall. You will immediately see the difference!

Although emphasis was initially placed on the presence of diverticula and pain on graded compression of the left lower quadrant, bowel wall thickness and hyperechoic fat stranding have been recently integrated in the diagnostic criteria for acute diverticulitis.

As always in visceral US, identification of landmarks is essential for not getting lost. Start by placing your probe transversally on the anterior axillary line. You need to search for and detect the following structures: the anterior superior iliac spine (ASIS), the iliac wing, and the iliac muscle immediately medial to the ASIS. The first hollow viscus you encounter sliding medially the probe should be the colon: it appears like an artifact of air and a blur acoustic shadow inside an oval/round-shaped visceral structure (Fig. 5.1). If you are lucky, you will soon recognize the typical wall stratification and only a few artifacts in the lumen (air and feces). However, most frequently you can only guess the colon thanks to the air artifacts.

Gently sliding the probe up and down, and gradually compressing the colon, your perception becomes a certainty due to the displacement of the air in the bowel

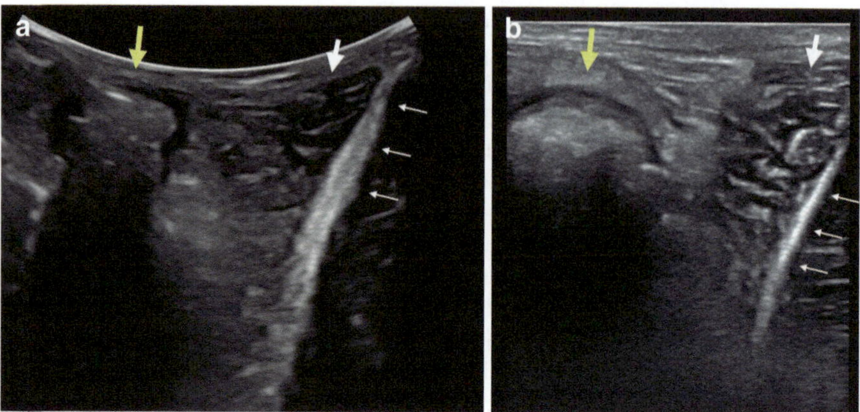

Fig. 5.1 Landmarks for US scanning of left colon ((**a**) convex probe; (**b**) linear probe). From left to right: ASIS and iliac bone (*light white arrows*), iliac muscle (*bold white arrow*), and large bowel in transversal view (*yellow arrow*). Note the better definition of the image with the linear probe: stratification of the bowel wall is clearly detectable

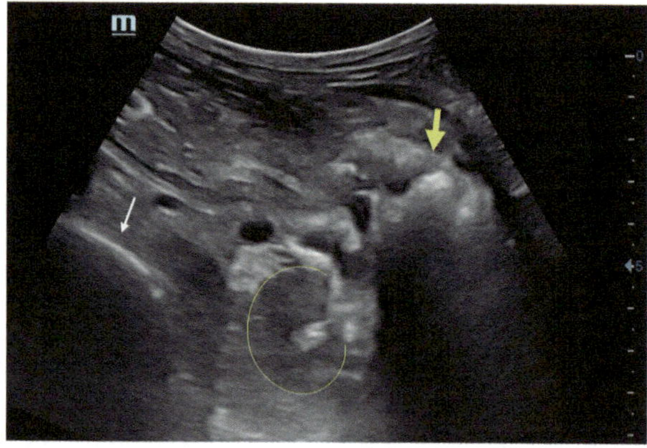

Fig. 5.2 Transversal view with a convex probe of the left kidney (*yellow curved line*) and the left colon (*yellow arrow*). Medially, a spine body with a complete shadow (*white arrow*)

lumen. But if you perceive an active peristalsis, you are probably wrong! Colonic peristalsis is not easily detected by US, so you are probably looking at a small bowel loop. Go back to your landmarks and restart the scan.

The large bowel is scanned in both the long and the short axis, following the diseased segment from normal anatomy towards pathological findings ("probe down" technique). The advice is to start far from the painful area, generally in the left flank, scanning first the descending colon, and thereafter sliding down the probe. Do first the scan of the colon in the short axis: if you maintain your target in the middle of the screen while sliding down the probe, it will be easier to follow the entire descending colon and the sigmoid colon, whatever the shape of the sigmoid loop would be. A longitudinal scan (long axis) could be useful only near the pelvis and when you get a possible paracolic abscess.

Are you still in trouble and can't find the colon? There is a last trick: ask the patient to turn on his/her right side. In the right lateral decubitus, the small bowel loops will fall to the right, whereas the left colon is fixed and will not fall. Again, do your scan transversally and search for the left kidney (transversal view) and the left colon (Fig. 5.2). Found it? Now, do not miss the view, hold the probe, and ask the patient to lie down again in the supine position: you should be ready for starting the "probe down" scan as described above.

Generally, the normal sonographic appearance of the bowel wall resembles the histological layers and is characterized by five alternating bands with different echogenicity ("gut signature"). In case of diverticulosis, the muscularis layer is often markedly thickened (>4 mm) and thin-walled diverticula can be easily recognized as round, echogenic, structures protruding in a relatively hyperechoic texture from the contracted colon. However, if the colon is filled with feces, the diverticula are difficult to be identified.

Diverticula of the left colon are usually acquired, false diverticula, lacking the muscularis propria. When scanning even with high-frequency probes, the wall of diverticula is substantially undetectable. Conversely, diverticula of the right colon are usually congenital, true diverticula, containing all bowel layers. They tend to be solitary, with a wide neck and no hypertrophy of the muscular layer. In both cases, a central shadowing echogenicity may indicate the presence of a fecalith.

In case of inflammation, the bowel wall becomes thickened, the pericolic fat increases its echogenicity, and pain is provoked by focused compression. This is a key point to remember, which makes the difference with other imaging techniques!

To simplify, here are two different scenarios:

- Painful sigmoid loop at graded compression, normal appearance of the colonic wall, no evidence of diverticula nor abscesses: depending on clinical presentation, it could be an infectious or not specific colitis, or it may be a simple fit of irritable bowel disease.
- Painful sigmoid loop at graded compression, segmental thickened colonic wall with diverticula, hyperechoic pericolic fat, no abscesses: this is a Hinchey 0 diverticulitis.

Color-Doppler is in general of limited value, the US diagnosis rely on B-mode views. The inflamed diverticulum appears as an enlarged hypoechoic sack protruding from the colonic wall, with loss of the gut signature and surrounded by echogenic fat, which represents the inflamed mesentery and/or omentum trying to wall off the pending perforation.

5.3 Clinical Meanings of Abnormal Findings

The main US features of an acutely inflamed diverticular bowel are wall thickness greater than 4 mm, pain on graded compression in the left iliac fossa, pericolic fat changes (more typically on the mesenteric side of the colonic wall) and the presence of diverticula. US can also detect the complications of diverticulitis, such as intra-abdominal-free fluid, free air, and abscesses.

One of the pathognomonic signs of acute diverticulitis was first described in 1985 by Parulekar, who reported a case series of 16 patients and illustrated the "pseudo-kidney" sign, which consists in a "target" appearance of the diseased colon, resulting from the inflamed concentric hypoechoic wall with a hyperechoic center determined by the reflections of mucosa and debris. However, more subtle changes may be present on US examination and their interpretation cannot preclude an accurate evaluation of the whole clinical context, including the patient history, physical examination, and laboratory findings.

When performing US, the clinician needs to be aware of potential differential diagnoses. For example, Crohn's disease may present with severe mural thickening and associated lymphadenopathy, but these findings are mostly present in the terminal ileum and ascending colon. Ulcerative colitis may reveal submucosal thickening and increased vascularity on Doppler mode, while pseudomembranous colitis presents the characteristic hyperechoic mucosa determining the "accordion sign appearance," similarly to CT scan. Unlike acute diverticulitis, colonic malignancy determines a distortion of the bowel wall architecture, and the tumor may be bulky and hyperechoic. The additional presence of liver metastases and pathological enlarged lymph nodes can also be quite suggestive of the diagnosis.

The key US features of acute diverticulitis are described below and summarized in Table 5.2. These are the most important features to be looked for when performing a targeted examination for suspected acute diverticulitis.

- **Thickened hypoechoic wall**: US shows transmural, circumferential, hypoechoic wall thickening of more than 4 mm on transverse view (Fig. 5.3), or up to 4 cm on longitudinal view, corresponding to the hypertrophy of the external circular muscle layer. According to Lembcke and colleagues, bowel wall thickening is a mandatory sign for diagnosis of acute diverticulitis and may be accompanied by a central hyperechoic area in about 40% of cases (i.e., "pseudo-kidney" sign).
- **Hyperechoic pericolic fat tissue** ("fat stranding"): the inflammatory process determines an increased vascularity in the pericolic and/or omental fat, which will appear as hyperechoic and non-compressible areas surrounding the thickened colon segment (Fig. 5.3).
- **Severe pain on graded compression**: focal tenderness induced by graded probe compression is a constant and important element of diagnosis, and it is produced

Table 5.2 US findings of acute colonic diverticulitis

Direct signs	Additional signs
Thickened wall (≥4 mm) **Detection of diverticula (with or without fecalith)** **Hyperechoic pericolic fat** **Pericolic abscess** **Pain at graded compression (with + signs)**	Distant free fluid (*possible H3/H4*) Pericolic trapped free air artifacts (*micro-perforation*) Distant abscess

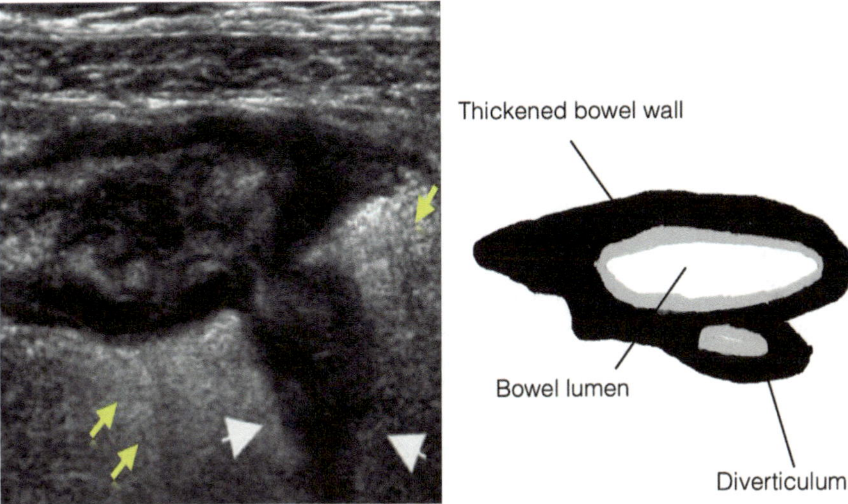

Fig. 5.3 Transverse US view of a thickened hypoechoic large bowel loop (*left*) and its graphic representation (*right*), outlining the US findings. The thickened bowel wall and the diverticulum (*white arrows*) can be seen. Hyperechoic brighter areas (*yellow arrows*) around the bowel lumen represent fat stranding

by the acute inflammatory process involving the bowel wall (analogous to what happens in acute appendicitis).

- **Detection of diverticula**: sometimes described as "dog ears," an inflamed diverticulum appears as a hypoechoic rim outpouching away from the colonic wall with loss of layering and surrounded by a "mesenteric cap." Acoustic shadowing behind a short white convex artifact is due to the presence of a fecalith (thickened feces) inside a diverticulum (Fig. 5.4). This finding can really help detecting a diverticulum and should be carefully distinguished from a pericolic abscess containing gas bubbles (in this latter case, shadowing is inconstant, tiny, and soft). Fecaliths could sometimes be detected even in asymptomatic diverticular disease and are not themselves a marker of acute diverticulitis.
- Although apparent in only 50% of cases, the fecalith presence increases the sensitivity of US in uncomplicated disease from 77% to 96%, with an overall accuracy of 86%. In complicated disease, the inflamed diverticulum will not be easily identified as the phlegmonous process and/or gangrene will obliterate it. In right-sided diverticulitis, the US evidence of inflamed diverticula may be the only diagnostic feature. As in the right colon diverticula are usually congenital, all bowel wall layers will be present, with no hypertrophy of the colonic wall.

Other additional US features that may help in the diagnosis of acute diverticulitis are:

- **Luminal narrowing and loss of compressibility**: as for acute appendicitis, the inflamed thickened bowel does not move and is not compressible.

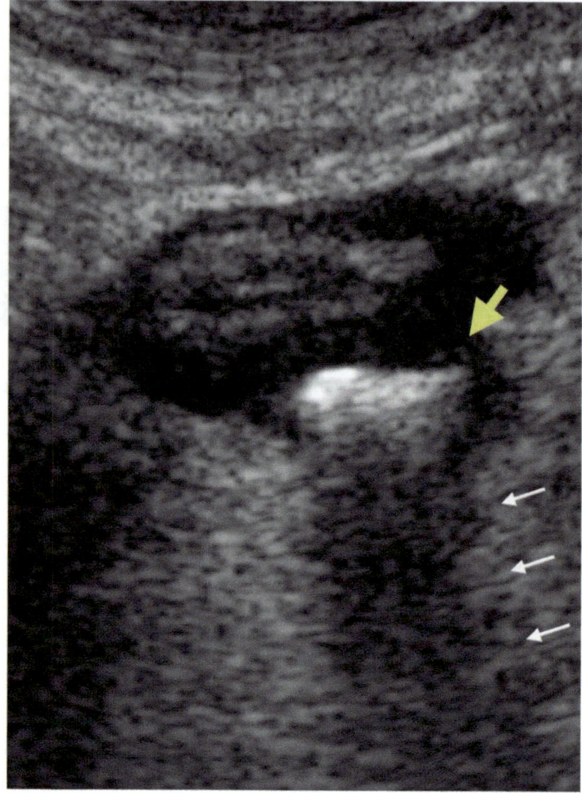

Fig. 5.4 US transverse section of a sigmoid acute diverticulitis with fecalith: hypoechoic thickened bowel wall, slightly hyperechoic pericolic fat, and detection of a fecalith. The latter is easily recognized as a hyperechoic spot inside a diverticulum (*yellow arrow*), determining an acoustic shadow (*white arrows*)

- **Intramural or pericolic abscess**: typically appearing as well-defined hypoechoic cystic mass with hyperechoic debris adjacent to the inflamed bowel segment (Fig. 5.5). Detection may be difficult when the collection is smaller than 2.5 cm in diameter, present gas inclusions, or is located between bowel loops.
- **Identification of fistula**: sometimes, a paracolic abscess may evacuate through the bladder, vagina (in females), or skin, determining the formation of a fistula. In these cases, the presence of gas can be identified within the target organ and the passage of gas bubbles could be witnessed from time to time.
- **Intra-abdominal-free fluid**: it is usually found between the bowel loops, in the left paracolic gutter, and/or in pelvis. A small amount of pericolic or pelvic fluid is not enough for defining a Hinchey 3 diverticulitis. Free fluid in the Morrison pouch, in paracolic gutters, or perisplenic is worrisome and must be coupled with the clinical status. A US-guided aspiration (DPA) can shorten the decision-making process, giving you an immediate information about the color (and the nature) of the fluid.
- **Increased vascularity on Color-Doppler mode**: assessment of bowel wall vasculature can be useful as, in case of acute inflammation, the bowel segment will

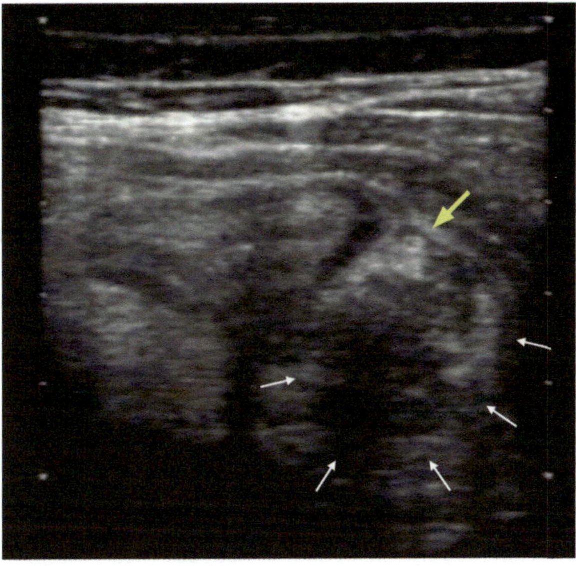

Fig. 5.5 Pericolic abscess (Hinchey 1B). Laterally to the transversal view of the large bowel, the hypoechoic area (*white arrows*) of about 25 mm (*look at the markers on the right side*) is well detectable with the linear probe. White artifacts at the top of the area (*yellow arrow*) mean small air bubbles inside. Graded compression will be painful

present with increased blood flow through the colonic wall. However, this information is rarely decisive.

When to use US in the clinical work-up? The answer is very easy: *always*, as the first imaging option and an immediately available tool for confirming your clinical suspicion. Let's summarize why.

US features of acute diverticulitis have been described since the late 1980s and US and CT scanning have been frequently compared in literature. In 2008, Laméris and colleagues performed an impressive meta-analysis to investigate the diagnostic accuracy of graded compression US and CT in acute colonic diverticulitis. Overall, 6 US studies encompassing 630 patients and 8 CT studies encompassing 684 patients were included for the analysis. Diagnostic criteria were bowel wall thickening and pericolic fat inflammation, with no mention of the presence of diverticula. Reference values were surgical findings and clinical outcomes on follow-up. The results did not show any statistical difference between US and CT in terms of sensitivity and specificity although CT scanning was more likely to identify alternative diseases.

The same group subsequently published their results on the comparison of US and CT accuracy in common diagnoses causing acute abdominal pain. Although not specifically related to acute diverticulitis, the results of these studies are significant for daily practice as clinical examination was performed by surgical trainees and imaging was performed by radiology residents, which is far from the ideal research environment usually encompassing field experts. In their analyses, the Dutch group reported that although CT scan is the most sensitive imaging modality, US can reliably detect common conditions determining acute abdominal pain. Interestingly, a significant difference was found between trainees with less than 500 US examinations performed and trainees with more than 500 US examinations performed. Moreover, US as a single test could miss over 30% of urgent conditions, whereas performing CT in equivocal cases would bring down the miss rate to 6%. Therefore, the authors concluded that US could be used as first imaging modality for patients presenting with acute abdominal pain, regardless of its origin, reserving CT for inconclusive or negative findings.

Based on the conditional strategy proposed by Laméris group, in 2014 Andeweg and colleagues proposed a step-up approach, where CT is performed only after an inconclusive or negative US examination. Under these circumstances, performing US as a first imaging investigation allows for the best sensitivity and lowers unnecessary exposure to radiations in acute uncomplicated diverticulitis.

Our own studies demonstrated a high sensitivity and a high specificity for US in detecting acute diverticulitis. We also confirmed that the clinical staging for mild degrees of the acute disease could be reliably assessed by US with an accuracy similar to CT, thus enhancing the possibility of safely establishing an outpatient treatment (Figs. 5.6 and 5.7).

However, CT is still essential when the "unhappy triad of intestinal ultrasound," as described by Zielke and colleagues (i.e., "too much fat, too much gas, or too much pain"), is encountered. Moreover, US should always be associated to a CT scan when clinical examination and location of pain suggest a pelvic extension of the acute diverticulitis (e.g., pelvic abscess, distal sigmoid inflammation), as US cannot accurately rule out a complicated disease.

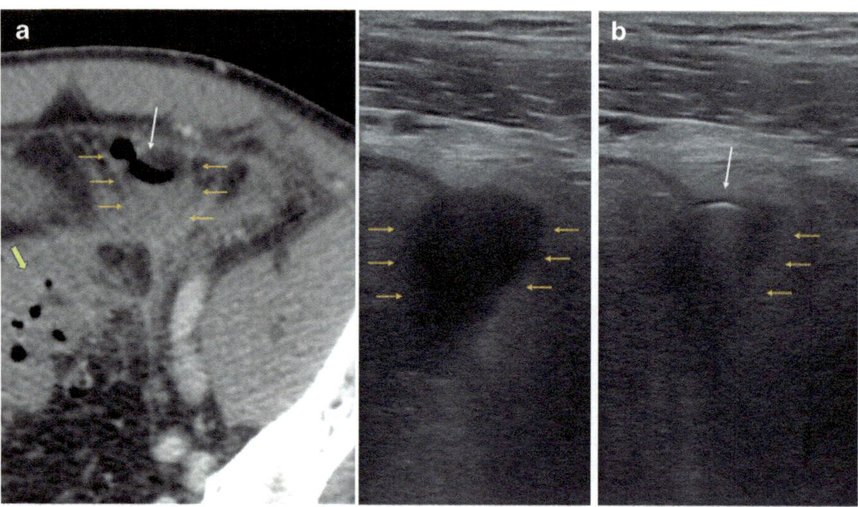

Fig. 5.6 Pericolic abscess (Hinchey 1B). There is a strict correspondence between CT findings (*on the left*) and US findings (*on the right*, **a** and **b**). Above the thickened sigmoid (*yellow arrow*), a paracolic abscess is clearly visible (*orange arrows*) on both CT and US pictures (linear probe). The air bubbles inside the abscess (*white arrow*) are detected on US imaging by slowly tilting the probe (**b**)

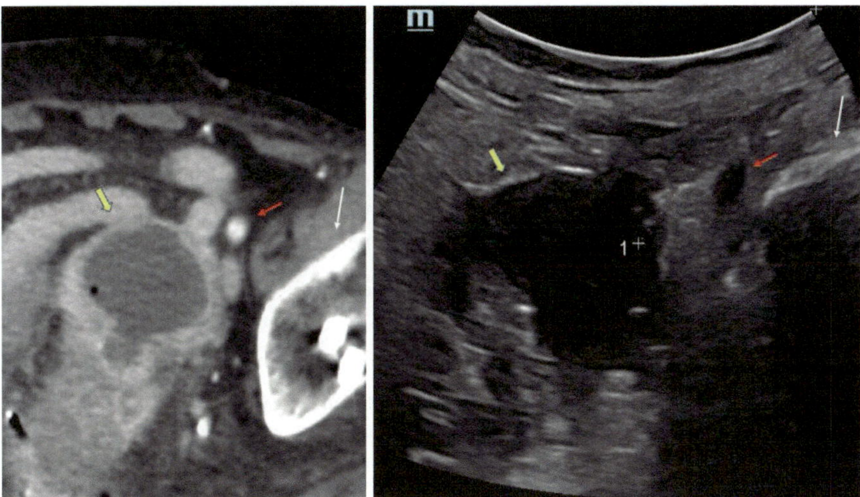

Fig. 5.7 Pelvic abscess (Hinchey 2). Strict correspondence between CT (*left*) and POCUS (*right*) pictures. The abscess (*yellow arrow*), the left iliac artery (*red arrow*), and the iliac bone (*white arrow*) are recognizable and symmetrically depicted. The dotted line marks the length and ideal path for an US-guided percutaneous drainage

US-guided aspiration and drainage of pericolic or distant abscesses are other demonstrations of possible US application in the field of acute complicated diverticulitis. However, their description is beyond the scope of this chapter.

Tips and Tricks

- Get the landmarks: antero-superior iliac spine, iliac muscle, and colon.
- Start scanning from the descending colon: as it is often not involved, you will not elicit pain.
- Measure the colonic wall.
- Wall thickening in case of sigmoid cancer is usually asymmetrical and moderately echogenic.

Red Flags

- **Warning**. A persistent, large paracolic abscess should always raise the suspicion of underlying malignancy.
- **Pitfall**. A fecalith at the base of a right colonic diverticulum may be mistaken for an inflamed appendix, leading to unnecessary operation.
- **Warning**. Perform US as a first imaging modality. However, in case of inconclusive or negative findings, do not hesitate to upgrade to a CT scan.

Appendix: Chapter 5—Test Yourself (Answers in the Appendix at the End of the Book)

Q1—A colonic diverticulum usually appears as …

- A hypoechoic round-shaped image surrounded by hyperechoic pericolic fat.
- A hyperechoic round-shaped image surrounded by hypoechoic pericolic fat.
- A dyshomogeneous hypo-/anechoic area near the colonic wall.

Q2—POCUS landmarks for finding the left colon are …?

- Colon, psoas muscle, iliac vessels.
- Bladder, iliac muscle, iliac vessels.
- ASIS, iliac muscle, descending/sigmoid colon.

Further Reading

Andeweg CS, Wegdam JA, Groenewoud J, van der Wilt GJ, van Goor H, Bleichrodt RP. Toward an evidence-based step-up approach in diagnosing diverticulitis. Scand J Gastroenterol. 2014;49(7):775–84. https://doi.org/10.3109/00365521.2014.908475.

Cuomo R, Barbara G, Pace F, Annese V, Bassotti G, Binda GA, et al. Italian consensus conference for colonic diverticulosis and diverticular disease. United Eur Gastroenterol J. 2014;2(5):413–42. https://doi.org/10.1177/2050640614547068.

Dumbrava BD, Abdulla HS, Pereira J, Biloslavo A, Zago M, Hashem JH, et al. Surgeon-performed point-of-care ultrasound in the diagnosis of acute sigmoid diverticulitis: a pragmatic prospective multicenter cohort study. Cureus. 2023;15(1):e33292. https://doi.org/10.7759/cureus.33292.

Helou N, Abdalkader M, Abu-Rustum RS. Sonography: first-line modality in the diagnosis of acute colonic diverticulitis? J Ultrasound Med. 2013;32(10):1689–94. https://doi.org/10.7863/ultra.32.10.1689.

Hollerweger A, et al. Gastrointestinal ultrasound (GIUS) in intestinal emergencies—an EFSUMB position paper Ultraschall in Med 2020; 41: 646–657 | © 2020. Thieme. All rights reserved.

King WC, Shuaib W, Vijayasarathi A, Fajardo CG, Cabrera WE, Costa JL. Benefits of sonography in diagnosing suspected uncomplicated acute diverticulitis. J Ultrasound Med. 2015;34(1):53–8. https://doi.org/10.7863/ultra.34.1.53.

Lembcke B. Diagnosis, differential diagnoses, and classification of diverticular disease. Viszeralmedizin. 2015;31(2):95–102. https://doi.org/10.1159/000380833.

Lembcke B. Ultrasonography in acute diverticulitis - credit where credit is due. Z Gastroenterol. 2016;54(1):47–57. https://doi.org/10.1055/s-0041-108204.

Lembcke BJ, Strobel D, Dirks K, Becker D, Menzel J. Statement of the section internal medicine of the DEGUM - ultrasound obtains pole position for clinical imaging in acute diverticulitis. Ultraschall Med. 2015;36(2):191–5. https://doi.org/10.1055/s-0034-1369761.

Laméris W, van Randen A, Bipat S, Bossuyt PM, Boermeester MA, Stoker J. Graded compression ultrasonography and computed tomography in acute colonic diverticulitis: meta-analysis of test accuracy. Eur Radiol. 2008;18(11):2498–511. https://doi.org/10.1007/s00330-008-1018-6.

Laméris W, van Randen A, van Es HW, van Heesewijk JP, van Ramshorst B, Bouma WH, et al. Imaging strategies for detection of urgent conditions in patients with acute abdominal pain: diagnostic accuracy study. BMJ. 2009;338:b2431. https://doi.org/10.1136/bmj.b2431.

Maconi G, Carmagnola S, Guzowski T. Intestinal ultrasonography in the diagnosis and management of colonic diverticular disease. J Clin Gastroenterol. 2016;50(Suppl 1):S20–2. https://doi.org/10.1097/MCG.0000000000000657.

Parulekar SG. Sonography of colonic diverticulitis. J Ultrasound Med. 1985;4(12):659–66. https://doi.org/10.7863/jum.1985.4.12.659.

Pradel JA, Adell JF, Taourel P, Djafari M, Monnin-Delhom E, Bruel JM. Acute colonic diverticulitis: prospective comparative evaluation with US and CT. Radiology. 1997;205(2):503–12. https://doi.org/10.1148/radiology.205.2.9356636.

Puylaert JB. Ultrasound of colon diverticulitis. Dig Dis. 2012;30(1):56–9. https://doi.org/10.1159/000336620.

Tham JC, Smolarek SK, Coleman MG. Diverticulitis, pelvic and other intra-abdominal abscesses. Surgery (Oxford). 2017;35:456–61. https://doi.org/10.1016/j.mpsur.2017.05.004.

Sartelli M, Catena F, Ansaloni L, Coccolini F, Griffiths EA, Abu-Zidan FM, et al. WSES Guidelines for the management of acute left sided colonic diverticulitis in the emergency setting. World J Emerg Surg. 2016;29(11):37. https://doi.org/10.1186/s13017-016-0095-0.

van Randen A, Laméris W, van Es HW, van Heesewijk HP, van Ramshorst B, Ten Hove W, et al. A comparison of the accuracy of ultrasound and computed tomography in common diagnoses causing acute abdominal pain. Eur Radiol. 2011;21(7):1535–45. https://doi.org/10.1007/s00330-011-2087-5.

Wasvary H, Turfah F, Kadro O, Beauregard W. Same hospitalization resection for acute diverticulitis. Am Surg. 1999;65(7):632–5; discussion 636.

Zago M, Biloslavo A, Mariani D, Pestalozza MA, Poillucci G, Bellio G. Surgeon-performed ultrasound for the staging of acute diverticulitis: Preliminary results of a prospective study. J Trauma Acute Care Surg. 2021;91(2):393–8. https://doi.org/10.1097/TA.0000000000003229.

Zielke A, Hasse C, Nies C, Kisker O, Voss M, Sitter H, et al. Prospective evaluation of ultrasonography in acute colonic diverticulitis. Br J Surg. 1997;84(3):385–8.

Chapter 6
Acute Appendicitis and US: A Never-Ending Story?

Diego Mariani, Isidro Martinez Casas, Andrea Casamassima, Antonio Rodrigues da Silva, Alexander Natroshvili, and Mauro Zago

6.1 Introduction

Acute appendicitis is one of the most common abdominal surgical emergencies, with a lifetime risk of about 7%. It usually affects children and young adults, but it can occur at any age. Characteristic presentation includes abdominal pain, starting

Supplementary Information The online version contains supplementary material available at https://doi.org/10.1007/978-3-031-40231-9_6.

D. Mariani (✉)
Department of General Surgery, ASST Ovest Milanese, "Ospedale Nuovo" di Legnano, Legnano, Milan, Italy

I. Martinez Casas
Department of General and Digestive Surgery, Virgen del Rocío University Hospital, Seville, Spain

A. Casamassima
Department of General Surgery, ASST Melegnano-Martesana, "Santa Maria delle Stelle" Hospital, Melzo, Milan, Italy

A. R. da Silva
Department of Surgery, Division of Colorectal Surgery, Hospital Pedro Hispano, Matosinhos, Portugal

A. Natroshvili
Sechenov First Moscow State Medical University, Sechenov University, Moscow, Russia

M. Zago
General and Emergency Surgery Unit, General Surgery Department, ASST Lecco, "A. Manzoni" Hospital, Lecco, Italy

M. Zago et al. (eds.), *Point-of-care US for Acute Abdomen*, https://doi.org/10.1007/978-3-031-40231-9_6

in periumbilical area and then migrating in the right iliac fossa, associated with nausea, vomiting, and fever. However, not all patients present in a typical manner, and diagnosis can be quite challenging, depending on patients age and anatomical position of the appendix. Despite the technological improvements and possibility of using dedicated scores (e.g., Alvarado score, Pediatric Appendicitis Score, Appendicitis Inflammatory Risk score, Adult Appendicitis Score, Ripasa score), no specific diagnostic test exists, and diagnosis is still predominantly clinical. A thorough history and physical examination are of paramount importance, as the only constant sign is acute or subacute abdominal pain. Antibiotics alone can be used in the early phase of acute appendicitis, but medical treatment is associated with relatively high recurrence rates, and surgical appendectomy remains the treatment of choice. Even so, acute appendicitis is still often misdiagnosed, and the reported rates of negative appendectomy can be as high as 15–30%.

Although the main aim remains to prevent complicated acute appendicitis by performing early operation, the morbidity and costs associated with negative appendectomy are not irrelevant and increasing evidence has demonstrated that preoperative imaging can reduce unnecessary intervention. In this context, ultrasonography (US) is the preferred initial imaging modality in the diagnosis of acute appendicitis. Although computed tomography (CT) and magnetic resonance imaging (MRI) are more sensitive and specific, the lower costs of US, as well as its broad availability, dynamic features, and lack of ionizing radiation, make it a particularly appealing imaging modality.

The effectiveness of US in the diagnosis of acute appendicitis was first reported by Puylaert in 1986, who described the technique known as *graded compression*. By using a linear probe over the site of maximal tenderness, as indicated by the patient, a gradual increasing pressure is exerted to displace disturbing bowel gas artifacts and reduce the distance between the transducer and the retroperitoneal structures, allowing for a more accurate visualization of the pathologic process.

Over the following decades, this technique has been extensively studied and was found to have satisfactory sensitivity and specificity both in the pediatric and adult populations (Table 6.1).

Although data varies across literature, it is widely accepted that US is an effective first-line diagnostic tool in patients with suspected acute appendicitis. However, US can be limited by the patient's anatomy, body habitus, and amount of bowel gas potentially obstructing the view. In case of negative and/or equivocal US results, clinical reassessment, as well as complementary imaging (i.e., CT scan and/or MRI), should be carried out.

Table 6.1 Positive predictive value (PPV) and negative predictive value (NPV) for clinical examination, CT scan, and compression US (adapted from *Toorenvliet et al.*, World J Surg 2010; 34:2278–2285)

	PPV (%)	NPV (%)
Clinical examination	63	98
CT scan	100	100
Compression US	94	97

The purpose of this chapter is to provide the most typical and atypical US features and let the reader familiarize with the use of compressive US as a complementary tool in the evaluation of patients with suspected acute appendicitis.

6.2 Scanning Technique

One of the biggest challenges of US imaging for acute appendicitis is to actually find the appendix! Once positively identified, assessing its normality or pathological features is relatively simple.

The appendix is a blind-ending tubular structure of variable length (8–10 cm on average), arising from the posteromedial border of the cecum, close to the ileocecal valve, and containing all layers of the colonic wall. Although the location of the base is quite constant, the tip can be variably situated. Apart from the so-called usual position, crossing iliac vessels in right iliac fossa, it could be retrocecal, subcecal, pre-ileal, post-ileal, pelvic, or subhepatic. This is important to know, because visualization of the appendix in its entirety is required, as acute inflammation may only affect the apex.

The examination begins with the patient in the supine position. For ease of compressibility, sometimes the abdominal wall musculature can be relaxed by having the patient bend the knees (but this position could fight with the examiner's arm). If necessary, provide pain medication before starting the examination.

Either linear high-frequency or curvilinear low-frequency probes can be used to detect the appendix. We recommend starting the examination using a low-frequency convex probe (3.5 MHz) in order to have a first general view of the entire abdomen, searching for free fluid and other possible concurrent diagnoses (like gynecological disorders in females). Thereafter, you can shift to the high-frequency linear probe (7.5 MHz), for a focused assessment of the appendix. At times, in obese patients, the examination might be possible only with the convex probe.

There are two possible "protocols" for getting the appendix: *top-to-down* (i.e., ascending colon—cecum—appendix) and *bottom-to-up* (i.e., iliac vessels—last bowel loop–cecum–appendix). The latter is advised for beginners and for those who find themselves quite lost looking at the "grey fog" in the right iliac fossa. In any case, the top five landmarks you need to recognize are reported in Table 6.2.

Top-to-Down Protocol Place the linear probe laterally in the right lower quadrant and slide it medially and downward, from the right anterior superior iliac spine

Table 6.2 US landmarks for appendix

Abdominal wall
Cecum
Terminal ileum
Psoas muscle
Iliac vessels

(ASIS) to the hypogastrium. Between the ASIS and the right psoas muscle, there is a visceral structure containing gas and fluid, representing the ascending colon and cecum. Moving the transducer down into the pelvis, always with a graded, intermittent, and gentle compression, identify the right iliac vessels. Keeping these landmarks in view, swing the probe up and down (*move the wrist only!*) along the border of the cecum, searching for the basis/body of the appendix.

Bottom-to-Up Protocol Place the linear probe transversally over the femoral vessels, at the groin. Slide up the probe, maintaining the iliac vessels in the middle of the screen. Do not compress the abdominal wall; the psoas muscle is on the left. At a certain point, a small bowel loop should appear. Slightly compress it to confirm it is the last bowel loop; by moving the probe on the right, follow its long axis and get to the cecum, filled by feces and gas. You are now in the right area: tilt and fan the probe, searching for the appendix. Pain complained by the patient can help you getting your target (and the target sign!).

Alternatively, you can also place the probe directly over the point of maximal tenderness as indicated by one finger of the patient (*be gentle!*) and identify the right psoas and iliac vessels by graded compression. The appendix usually lies just anterior to these structures, behind the last small bowel loop. Once identified, confirm that it is the appendix by visualizing it in both the transverse (Fig. 6.1a) and longitudinal (Fig. 6.1b) axis.

Remember that graded compression allows to move the bowel gas out of the US plane and to bring the appendix closer to the abdominal wall. A normal appendix is generally less than 6 mm in diameter, not compressible (*as always*), not painful, without peristalsis (*as always*), and surrounded by homogeneous fat. In case of inflammation, the appendix becomes a sausage-like, non-compressible structure that lacks peristalsis and appears concentrically layered (“target” sign), with possible increased vascularization of the wall and surrounding fat. Focused graded compression will usually elicit a variable amount of pain.

6.3 Abnormal Findings

Table 6.3 summarize the direct and indirect US finding for the diagnosis of acute appendicitis.

Primary findings in case of acute appendicitis are required for achieving a high specificity. They all entail direct visualization of the appendix. Note that graded compression over the appendix allows you to obtain two of them:

- ***Outer diameter >6 mm***: the size of the appendix is one of the most important diagnostic criteria for acute appendicitis. It is generally accepted that the maximal outer diameter of a normal appendix does not exceed 6 mm on a transversal view. A size exceeding 6 mm is both 95% sensitive and specific for acute appendicitis. The thickness of the appendiceal wall is not diagnostic.

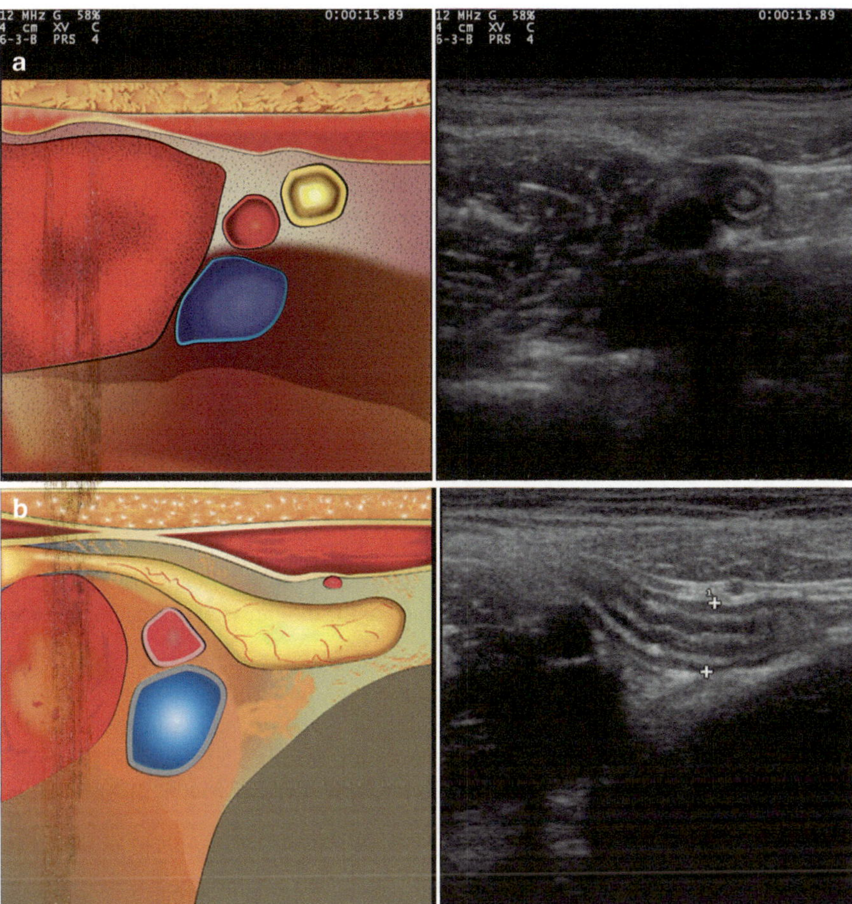

Fig. 6.1 (**a**) Identification of the appendix and its landmarks—transverse axis. Note the typical target sign of the appendix in its short axis. (**b**) Identification of the appendix and its landmarks—longitudinal axis

Table 6.3 Direct and indirect US criteria for the diagnosis of acute appendicitis

Direct signs	Indirect signs
Ø ≥ 6 mm	Peri-cecal free fluid/fluid collection/abscess
Non-compressible	Hyperechogenic surrounding fat
Pain on focused compression	Detection of appendicolith
Target sign (bull's eye)	Enlarged mesenteric lymph nodes
	Hypervascularized CFM pattern
	Thickening of cecum and distal ileum
	Dilation of adjacent bowel loops

- ***Non-compressibility***: the appendix is a blind-ending, tubular structure that, even under normal circumstances, is not (or very slightly) compressible. In case of inflammation, the edematous swelling of the wall determines full non-compressibility of the appendix. This is evident since the early stages of acute inflammation but can be lacking in case of perforation. The graded compression allows to differentiate the tubular structure deemed to be the appendix from a bowel loop, which is normally fully compressible and maintains a slight visible compressibility even in case of inflammation.
- ***Pain on compression***: this sign is pathognomonic, provided that the identified tubular structure is actually the appendix.
- ***Bull's eye sign (or target sign)***: as a true diverticulum, the appendix presents all layers of the colonic wall that are normally seen as alternating echogenic and hypoechoic concentric layers. As the appendix becomes swollen and inflamed, the US appearance on a transverse scan will be characterized by a hypoechoic center (i.e., the lumen filled with fluid), surrounded by a hyperechoic ring (i.e., inflamed mucosal and submucosal layers), surrounded by an outer hypoechoic ring (i.e., muscular layer). See Fig. 6.1a.

When the appendix is not directly visualized by point-of-care US (POCUS), secondary findings can help raise the accuracy of the diagnosis of acute appendicitis:

- ***Hyperechoic surrounding fat***: the fat tissues surrounding the appendix (i.e., the mesentery and the omentum trying to wall-off the inflammatory process) can become hyperechoic and non-compressible. This US feature corresponds to the fat stranding seen on CT scan. However, it is not specific, and it could be observed in other inflammatory processes (e.g., Crohn's disease, Meckel diverticulitis, ileitis).
- ***Free fluid or fluid collections***: small amount of intra-peritoneal fluid can be found in both complicated (i.e., perforated) and non-complicated acute appendicitis, as well as in patients with a normal appendix. Initially surrounding the appendix, with the evolving of the inflammatory process the fluid may be found around the cecum, in the right paracolic gutter, and in the pelvis. In the early stages, it appears hypoechoic, but echogenic floating particles and fibrin strands can be observed with the worsening of inflammation and infection of the peritoneum. Large echogenic collections, especially if adjacent to dilated, hypodynamic bowel loops, are highly suspicious for perforated appendicitis.
- ***Appendicolith(s)***: hyperechoic structure(s) with posterior acoustic shadowing within the lumen of the appendix. They are thought to be the cause of most cases of acute appendicitis and can be seen in up to 35% of cases.
- ***Enlarged mesenteric lymph nodes***: secondary enlarged lymph nodes can be found in case of acute appendicitis, as well as secondary to other inflammatory process (e.g., Crohn's disease, infectious ileocolitis). If enlarged (and painful on graded compression) nodes are the only US findings in a young patient with right lower quadrant pain, a viral mesenteric lymphadenitis should be considered in the differential diagnosis.

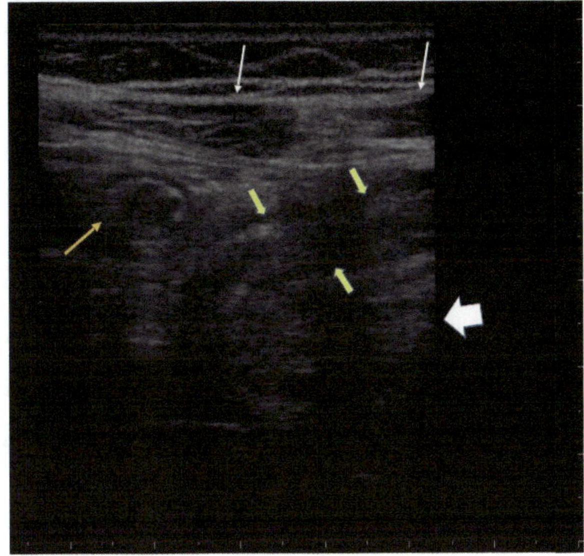

Fig. 6.2 Linear probe, transversal view. The rectus abdominis (*thin white arrows*), psoas (*bold white arrow*), small bowel loop on its short axis (*orange arrow*), and pathological appendix (*yellow arrows*). Note the caliper of the appendix, around 10 mm (look at the lateral grid on the right of the screen)

- ***Hypervascularization***: Color Doppler mode with Color Flow Mapping (CFM) can be a valuable adjunct to standard compressive US. In the early stages of acute inflammation, there may be no detectable increase in flow signal. However, as the inflammatory response increase, hypervascularization will be detected within the appendix wall and in the surrounding fat tissues. Anyway, this finding requires a high grade of experience and a perfect setting of CFM.
- ***Thickening of adjacent cecum and small bowel loops, dilation of adjacent small bowel loops, with loss of peristalsis***: these signs could mark a complicated appendicitis, identifying the so-called appendiceal mass.

Figures 6.2 and 6.3 show you some pathological images.

In 2015, Larson and colleagues published a prospective evaluation of over 1300 cases and proposed the adoption of a standardized structured appendix US report incorporating a five-category interpretive scheme according to US findings (Fig. 6.4). Interpretative categories were positive, dubious, or negative when the appendix was visualized, and secondary signs or no secondary signs when the appendix was not visualized. Overall, this approach determined a 97% accuracy for the diagnosis of acute appendicitis.

Remember that the most frequent alternative diagnosis in children is mesenteric lymphadenitis (Fig. 6.5).

Depending on age, sex, and comorbidities of the patient, alternative conditions potentially mimicking acute appendicitis should always be kept in mind when performing POCUS for suspected acute appendicitis. The main differential diagnoses are summarized in Table 6.4.

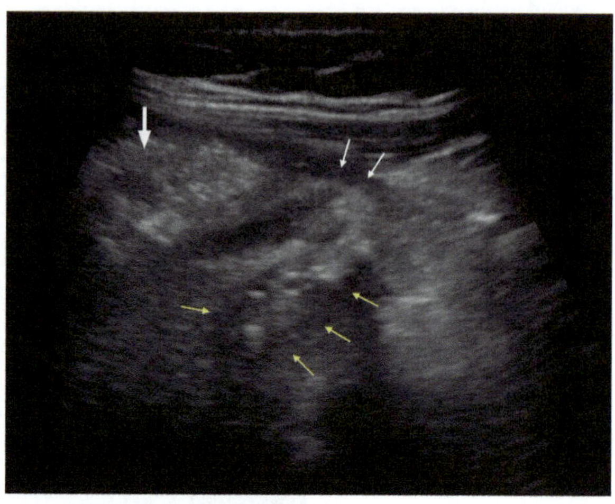

Fig. 6.3 Gangrenous appendicitis with normal appendiceal basis. The appendiceal basis (*thin white arrows*) emerges from the cecum (*bold white arrow*). The distal part of the appendix is enlarged, and painful on graded compression (*yellow arrows*). The small white spots inside the apex of the appendix suggest a gangrenous evolution

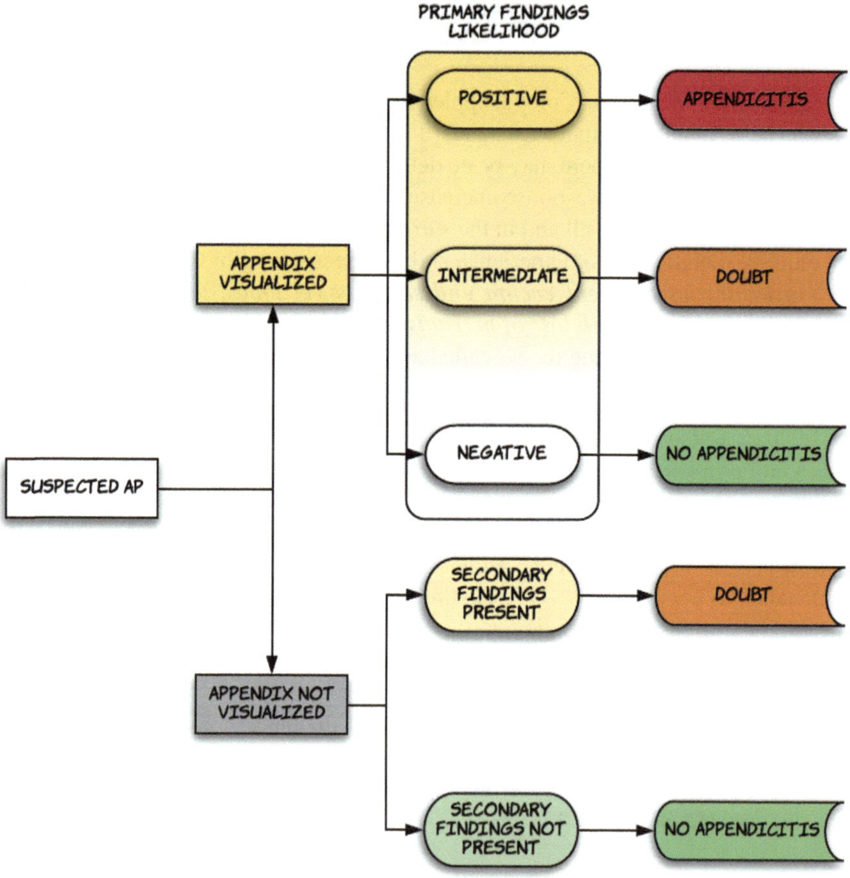

PRIMARY FINDINGS LIKELIHOOD

SUSPECTED AP

APPENDIX VISUALIZED

POSITIVE → APPENDICITIS

INTERMEDIATE → DOUBT

NEGATIVE → NO APPENDICITIS

APPENDIX NOT VISUALIZED

SECONDARY FINDINGS PRESENT → DOUBT

SECONDARY FINDINGS NOT PRESENT → NO APPENDICITIS

Fig. 6.4 US evaluation for acute appendicitis in children, according to a scheme incorporating equivocal diagnoses (derived from *Larson et al*, AJR Am J Roentgenol 2015; 204(4):849-856)

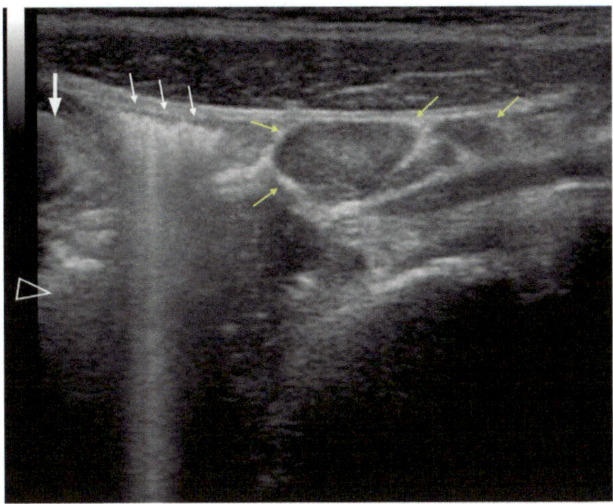

Fig. 6.5 Mesenteric adenitis. Behind the rectus muscle, from the left, identify the cecum (*bold arrow*), the psoas muscle (*empty arrow*), a small bowel loop with air artifacts (*thin white arrows*), and an enlarged lymph node (*yellow arrows*). A smaller lymph node is detectable medially. Painful lymph nodes at graded compression with normal or not visualized appendix are quite pathognomonic of mesenteric adenitis

Table 6.4 Differential diagnosis for suspected acute appendicitis

Inflammatory bowel disease (e.g., Crohn's disease, ulcerative colitis Invagination Small bowel diverticulitis Right-sided colonic diverticulitis, sigmoid diverticulitis Meckel's diverticulum (complications) Mesenteric lymphadenitis Invagination Volvulus Epiploic appendagitis Bowel ischemia Omental infarction	Ileocecal tuberculosis Infectious ileocolitis Neoplastic processes Gynecologic conditions (e.g., ruptured ovarian cyst, pelvic inflammatory disease, ovarian torsion, ectopic pregnancy, endometriosis, tubo-ovarian abscess) Urolithiasis (e.g., ureteral stones, pyelonephritis) Acute cholecystitis Duodenal ulcer Right basal pneumonia

Tips and Tricks

- Put the probe where it hurts, as indicated by the patient (but start far from this point, like in every clinical examination!). It usually helps expediting the evaluation.
- Don't be afraid of applying pressure, but do it in a gentle and graded fashion, so not to cause excessive pain.
- Compression allows to squeeze gas and bowel contents. Once the air has been displaced, slide the probe while continuing to gradually compress every 10 s, to prevent re-accumulation of gas in the visualized segment.
- Ask the patient to flex the legs a little, to relax the abdominal wall musculature and ease the compression.
- In case of troubles at visualizing the appendix, place the patient on a left lateral decubitus.
  - In this way, the small bowel loops will move out of the US plane and the appendix will appear anterior to the right psoas muscle on the screen.
  - If still not visualized, return the patient to the supine position for another attempt.
- The left lateral decubitus could allow you to search for a retrocecal appendicitis as well.

Red Flags

- **Pitfall**: be patient and always identify your landmarks (sequence ASIS, right psoas muscle, right iliac vessels).
- **Warning**: if POCUS is equivocal or negative, acute appendicitis cannot be ruled out without further evidence.

Appendix: Chapter 6—Test Yourself (Answers in the Appendix at the End of the Book)

Q1—The maximum normal diameter of the appendix is …?
5 mm
8 mm
6 mm
Q2—POCUS landmarks for acute appendicitis are …?
Bladder, psoas muscle, iliac vessels
Cecum, psoas, iliac vessels, distal ileum

ASIS, psoas, ascending colon

Further Reading

Andersson RE. Routine ultrasound and limited computed tomography for the diagnosis of acute appendicitis: a surgeon's perspective. World J Surg. 2011;35(2):295–6. https://doi.org/10.1007/s00268-010-0866-9.

Cohen B, Bowling J, Midulla P, Shlasko E, Lester N, Rosenberg H, et al. The non-diagnostic ultrasound in appendicitis: is a non-visualized appendix the same as a negative study? J Pediatr Surg. 2015;50(6):923–7. https://doi.org/10.1016/j.jpedsurg.2015.03.012.

Estey A, Poonai N, Lim R. Appendix not seen: the predictive value of secondary inflammatory sonographic signs. Pediatr Emerg Care. 2013;29(4):435–9. https://doi.org/10.1097/PEC.0b013e318289e8d5.

Gwynn LK. The diagnosis of acute appendicitis: clinical assessment versus computed tomography evaluation. J Emerg Med. 2001;21(2):119–23. https://doi.org/10.1016/s0736-4679(01)00353-5.

Humes DJ, Simpson J. Acute appendicitis. BMJ. 2006;333(7567):530–4. https://doi.org/10.1136/bmj.38940.664363.AE.

Larson DB, Trout AT, Fierke SR, Towbin AJ. Improvement in diagnostic accuracy of ultrasound of the pediatric appendix through the use of equivocal interpretive categories. AJR Am J Roentgenol. 2015;204(4):849–56. https://doi.org/10.2214/AJR.14.13026.

Noguchi T, Yoshimitsu K, Yoshida M. Periappendiceal hyperechoic structure on sonography: a sign of severe appendicitis. J Ultrasound Med. 2005;24(3):323–7; quiz 328–30. https://doi.org/10.7863/jum.2005.24.3.323.

Puylaert JB. Acute appendicitis: US evaluation using graded compression. Radiology. 1986;158(2):355–60. https://doi.org/10.1148/radiology.158.2.2934762.

Quigley AJ, Stafrace S. Ultrasound assessment of acute appendicitis in paediatric patients: methodology and pictorial overview of findings seen. Insights Imaging. 2013;4(6):741–51. https://doi.org/10.1007/s13244-013-0275-3.

Rettenbacher T, Hollerweger A, Macheiner P, Rettenbacher L, Tomaselli F, Schneider B, et al. Outer diameter of the vermiform appendix as a sign of acute appendicitis: evaluation at US. Radiology. 2001;218(3):757–62. https://doi.org/10.1148/radiology.218.3.r01fe20757.

Ross MJ, Liu H, Netherton SJ, Eccles R, Chen PW, Boag G, et al. Outcomes of children with suspected appendicitis and incompletely visualized appendix on ultrasound. Acad Emerg Med. 2014;21(5):538–42. https://doi.org/10.1111/acem.12377.

Shah BR, Stewart J, Jeffrey RB, Olcott EW. Value of short-interval computed tomography when sonography fails to visualize the appendix and shows otherwise normal findings. J Ultrasound Med. 2014;33(9):1589-1595. doi: https://doi.org/10.7863/ultra.33.9.1589. Erratum in: J Ultrasound Med. 2015 Jul;34(7):1300. Jeffery, R Brooke [corrected to Jeffrey, R Brooke].

Shogilev DJ, Duus N, Odom SR, Shapiro NI. Diagnosing appendicitis: evidence-based review of the diagnostic approach in 2014. West J Emerg Med. 2014;15(7):859–71. https://doi.org/10.5811/westjem.2014.9.21568.

Toorenvliet BR, Wiersma F, Bakker RF, Merkus JW, Breslau PJ, Hamming JF. Routine ultrasound and limited computed tomography for the diagnosis of acute appendicitis. World J Surg. 2010;34(10):2278–85. https://doi.org/10.1007/s00268-010-0694-y.

Trout AT, Towbin AJ, Fierke SR, Zhang B, Larson DB. Appendiceal diameter as a predictor of appendicitis in children: improved diagnosis with three diagnostic categories derived from a logistic predictive model. Eur Radiol. 2015;25(8):2231–8. https://doi.org/10.1007/s00330-015-3639-x.

Chapter 7
Bowel Ischemia: When Can US Make the Difference?

Antonio La Greca, Alan Biloslavo, Jorge Pereira, Luis Pinheiro, Marina Troian, and Hayato Kurihara

7.1 Introduction

Bowel ischemia, also known as mesenteric ischemia or intestinal ischemia, is an abdominal emergency characterized by vascular compromise of the bowel and its mesentery. It represents about 2% of all causes of emergency department (ED) consultations, and it encompasses a wide variety of conditions that can be either acute or chronic and may involve the small bowel, the large bowel, or both. Most patients are over 50–60 years of age and clinical presentation may vary depending on the underlying cause. Generally, patients complain abdominal pain that in the acute setting is quite severe, disproportionate to examination findings, and poorly respond to pain killers. Other associated symptoms include nausea, vomiting, and diarrhea. In more advanced phases, patients will develop peritoneal signs, including abdominal

A. La Greca (✉)
Department of Medical and Surgical Sciences, Emergency Surgery Unit, IRCCS Fondazione Policlinico Universitario "A. Gemelli", Catholic University of the Sacred Heart, Rome, Italy
e-mail: antonio.lagreca@policlinicogemelli.it

A. Biloslavo
Department of General Surgery, ASUGI, Cattinara University Hospital, Trieste, Italy

J. Pereira · L. Pinheiro
Department of General Surgery, Centro Hospitalar Tondela-Viseu, Hospital São Teotónio, Viseu, Portugal

M. Troian
Cardiothoracic and Vascular Department, ASUGI Cattinara University Hospital, Trieste, Italy

H. Kurihara
Department of Emergency Surgery, Fondazione IRCCS Ca' Granda, Ospedale Maggiore Policlinico, Milan, Italy

M. Zago et al. (eds.), *Point-of-care US for Acute Abdomen*,
https://doi.org/10.1007/978-3-031-40231-9_7

distension and guarding, tachycardia, and hypotension. If not promptly treated, mortality can be very high (50–90%), depending on etiology, time passed from clinical onset, and extent of diseased bowel segments.

Acute ischemia is more common than chronic ischemia and can result from arterial occlusion (60–85%), venous occlusion (5–15%), non-occlusive mesenteric ischemia (NOMI, 15–30%), or mixed conditions (e.g., strangulated bowel obstruction). The impaired perfusion initially determines transient superficial changes in the mucosal layer. If the blood flow is not quickly restored, the pathological process progresses towards transmural bowel wall necrosis, bacteria proliferations with gas release within the bowel wall (i.e., *pneumatosis intestinalis*) and then through the mesenteric vessels into the portal vein system (i.e., *pneumatosis portalis*), sepsis, intestinal perforation, and ultimately death.

Contrast-enhanced computed tomography (CT) of the abdomen and pelvis is the investigation of choice for patients with suspected intestinal ischemia, as it can adequately assess the etiology, as well as the degree and length of ischemic bowel, with sensitivity and specificity of up to 96% and 94%, respectively. However, abdominal ultrasound (US) is becoming increasingly used as first examination of patients with acute abdomen. As it is widely available, non-invasive, and relatively inexpensive, US allows dynamic evaluation of the bowel and its surrounding structures with no radiation burden. However, the gastrointestinal tract cannot be visualized in its entire length, findings can be non-specific, and imaging interpretation depends on operator's experience. Moreover, it can be difficult to perform in the obese or poorly compliant patients or in case of excessive amount of air in the intestinal loops.

Despite these limitations, US has been shown to be a valuable imaging method in the acute setting of suspected bowel ischemia. According to Lopez and colleagues, US carries a high positive predictive value for the diagnosis of ischemic colitis in patients over 50 years of age presenting with sudden abdominal pain and/or rectal bleeding and in whom abdominal US shows a thickened segment of colon of more than 10 cm in length. Similarly, Hosokawa and colleagues showed that the presence of superior mesenteric artery collapse, ascites, and a large intestinal twist on US imaging of pediatric patients with suspected intestinal volvulus were significant predictors of intestinal ischemic changes, thus prompting immediate surgical intervention. Moreover, US examination can be enhanced by Doppler mode and/or contrast media that may show any occlusion in the superior mesenteric vessels and help assessing bowel wall perfusion even in the early phases of intestinal ischemia.

7.2 Scanning Technique

As already outlined in the previous chapters, imaging of the gastrointestinal tract requires both low and high frequency, high resolution, linear or convex probes, as well as a great deal of patience and scanning experience.

The ileocecal region and the sigmoid colon can be easily identified in most patients. Fundamental landmarks of these regions are the right and left iliac vessels, respectively. The remaining colonic segments and the small bowel can be assessed by continuous scanning.

The gastrointestinal tract has a typical multilayered sonographic appearance, resulting from its highly stratified histology. The colonic segments can be sometimes distinguished by the haustra, whereas the small intestine usually presents circular mucosal folds and more fluid contents. Any disruption in these patterns can aid in the diagnosis of bowel pathology.

In this context, the most important and reliable sign of bowel disease is bowel wall thickening. Under normal circumstances, the bowel measures no more than 2–3 mm in thickness when examined with graded compression in both the adult and pediatric population. In addition, the overall echo texture, as well as the appearance of surrounding structures (i.e., mesentery, omentum, lymph nodes) are of paramount importance in the interpretation of US findings. Decreased and/or altered bowel motility is a non-specific sign of unhealthy bowel, whereas abnormally echogenic fat surrounding a bowel tract may indicate an area that deserves closer examination.

Color and Power Doppler modes enhance standard grey-scale imaging by providing additional information on the vascularity of the bowel wall and mesentery. Although probably not sensitive, a diminished bowel wall vascularity is a specific sign of intestinal ischemia. Moreover, mesenteric Doppler US has been advocated as a potentially accurate modality for detection of high-grade superior mesenteric artery stenosis, with high sensitivity and high negative predictive value. Fine-tuning of both Color and Power Doppler functions on your US equipment is paramount for getting correct findings. However, this is out of the scope of this chapter, and it ideally requires a brief focused hands-on training.

Contrast-enhanced US (CEUS) is another valuable tool that can aid in the evaluation of visceral arteries, as well as of the microcirculation of the bowel and surrounding structures.

7.3 US Findings in Case of Bowel Ischemia

7.3.1 Acute Arterial Mesenteric Ischemia

In 60–85% of cases, acute mesenteric ischemia is caused by arterial embolism or thrombosis in the celiac trunk, superior mesenteric artery, inferior mesenteric artery, or their branches. Therefore, the impaired blood flow may affect all or portions of the small bowel, right colon, transverse colon, and left colon according to the distribution of the involved vessels.

In the early phases of bowel ischemia, US examination may show fluid-filled, spastic bowel loops, although an increased amount of intraluminal gas may cause an acoustic barrier. Doppler US and CEUS can show stenosis in the celiac trunk or mesenteric vessels, as well as a reduced blood flow within the bowel wall.

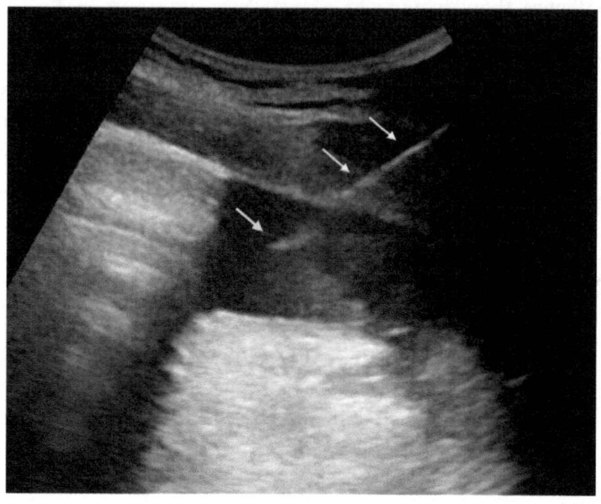

Fig. 7.1 US-guided DPA: the tip (*yellow arrow*) of the needle (*white arrows*) is clearly visible as a hyperechoic pointed structure

In the late phases, the bowel wall becomes thinner, and the loops appear fluid-filled with decreased/absent peristalsis and associated extraluminal fluid. This latter finding must be searched systematically whenever a bowel ischemia (arterial, venous, or NOMI) is suspected, entailing the option to perform a diagnostic peritoneal aspiration (DPA) for characterizing the nature of the fluid (Fig. 7.1). A serosanguineous fluid in the syringe is highly suspicious for transmural necrosis and mandate surgical exploration.

7.3.2 Acute Venous Mesenteric Ischemia

Venous mesenteric ischemia accounts for 5–15% of all cases of bowel ischemia and is determined by an occlusion in the territory of drainage of the superior mesenteric vein, with subsequent engorgement, swelling, and hemorrhage of the bowel wall and extravasation of fluids in the peritoneal cavity.

In the early phases, US may show bowel wall thickening and edema, characterized by echogenic mucosal layer and hypoechoic submucosal layer. Doppler mode and CEUS may reveal a thrombus in the superior mesenteric vein. With the progression of disease, the involved bowel segments will appear thickened, distended by intraluminal secretions, with decreased/absent movements and free extraluminal fluid. In the late stages, US may detect intramural gas and/or extraluminal free air.

7.3.3 Non-occlusive Mesenteric Ischemia

In 15–30% of cases, bowel ischemia can occur following a non-occlusive reduction of arterial blood blow, determining the so-called non-occlusive mesenteric ischemia (NOMI). In most patients, NOMI is characterized by primary vasoconstriction of the superior mesenteric artery and its branches, determining subsequent blood impairment in the small bowel and proximal colon. Early diagnosis requires a high index of clinical suspicion in patients with risk factors (*often these patients are in intensive care units*), and the condition is managed by reversal of eliciting factors, including—if possible—cessation of vasoconstrictive drugs and correction of the underlying cause of hypoperfusion.

In this setting, US findings can be quite non-specific, showing thinning of the bowel wall, decreased bowel movements, free fluid, and possible signs of parenchymal hypoperfusion. If the blood pressure is restored, reperfusion damage ensues with thickening of the bowel wall and gas-fluid mixed stasis. If the underlying cause is not timely resolved, the ischemic damage progresses, and US will show severe necrosis of the bowel wall, with intramural gas, extraluminal-free fluid, and fluid collections.

7.3.4 Ischemic Colitis

Ischemic colitis (IC) is the most frequent form of bowel ischemia and the second most frequent cause of lower gastrointestinal bleeding. It is characterized by an acute or, more commonly, chronic decrease in the blood flow of colonic wall small vessels, which may be either occlusive or, more often, non-occlusive in origin. Common risk factors include hypertension, ischemic heart disease, arteriosclerosis, diabetes mellitus, and age.

Clinical presentation varies from mild forms to fulminant cases. Most patients present with mild or transient disease, characterized by reversible lesions limited to the mucosal and submucosal layers, and benefit from conservative management, including hydration, antibiotic therapy, and correction of eliciting factors. Less frequently, IC may be characterized by a gangrenous form with transmural necrosis and high mortality, if not promptly recognized and treated.

The colon is typically affected in a segmental fashion, with the splenic flexure, descending colon, and sigmoid colon the most frequently involved segments. As demonstrated by Ripolles and colleagues, IC should be suspected in elderly patients with US findings of bowel wall thickening of a long colonic segment (>10 cm), especially on the left side, with barely visible or no color Doppler signal intensity. However, it is important to note that the absence of color Doppler flow is not sensitive, as it may be due to both technical (e.g., flow rate too low to be detected by available US equipment, incorrect tuning of color flow mapping on the equipment) and patient-related (e.g., body habitus, compliance during examination) variables. CEUS can help in differentiate ischemic from infectious colitis (see Chapter 10).

Although in most cases IC resolves spontaneously, it is important to identify those patients who may progress to complicated form of disease. Various clinical factors have been associated with IC outcomes, including patient age, length of affected bowel segment, concomitant cardiovascular disease, hypovolemic shock, and time passed from clinical onset and diagnosis.

On US examination, pericolic fat changes have been found to be predictive of transmural necrosis. However, none of these factors have been found to reliably predict the course of IC. Therefore, early diagnosis, close follow-up and prompt recognition of persistent disease are of paramount importance in the successful management of patients with IC.

Tips and Tricks

- Scan systematically. Use the convex probe first, then the linear one
- Mesenteric and omental fat are generally inconspicuous except when inflamed
  - Abnormal echogenic pericolic fat should prompt closer evaluation of the adjacent bowel segment as it can be predictive of transmural necrosis
- CEUS may provide useful information regarding mural and mesenteric blood flow, allowing for unequivocal diagnosis of visceral artery stenosis and bowel wall ischemia

Remember!

- *Pitfall*: absent or barely visible color Doppler flow is highly suggestive of ischemic thickening of the bowel wall although it may be limited by poor sensitivity for low flow rates, as well as by excessive abdominal fat or meteorism
- *Warning*: the presence of free peritoneal fluid should always suggest possible bowel disease until proven otherwise! However, it needs to be correlated with the whole clinical picture
- *Remember!* The absence of free peritoneal fluid does not exclude bowel disease
- *When in doubt*, perform diagnostic peritoneal aspiration (*DPA*). The linear probe allows you to find even small amount of fluid and to pick up a sample

Further Reading

Cavalcoli F, Zilli A, Fraquelli M, Conte D, Massironi S. Small bowel ultrasound beyond inflammatory bowel disease: an updated review of the recent literature. Ultrasound Med Biol. 2017;43(9):1741–52. https://doi.org/10.1016/j.ultrasmedbio.2017.04.028.

López E, Ripolles T, Martinez MJ, Bartumeus P, Blay J, López A. Positive predictive value of abdominal sonography in the diagnosis of ischemic colitis. Ultrasound Int Open. 2015;1(2):E41–5. https://doi.org/10.1055/s-0035-1,559,775.

Maturen KE, Wasnik AP, Kamaya A, Dillman JR, Kaza RK, Pandya A, et al. Ultrasound imaging of bowel pathology: technique and keys to diagnosis in the acute abdomen. AJR Am J Roentgenol. 2011;197(6):W1067–75. https://doi.org/10.2214/AJR.11.6594.

Medellin A, Merrill C, Wilson SR. Role of contrast-enhanced ultrasound in evaluation of the bowel. Abdom Radiol (NY). 2018;43(4):918–33. https://doi.org/10.1007/s00261-017-1399-6.

Pastor-Juan MDR, Ripollés T, Martí-Bonmatí L, Martínez MJ, Simó L, Gómez D, et al. Predictors of severity in ischemic colitis: usefulness of early ultrasonography. Eur J Radiol. 2017;96:21–6. https://doi.org/10.1016/j.ejrad.2017.09.003.

Reginelli A, Genovese E, Cappabianca S, Iacobellis F, Berritto D, Fonio P, et al. Intestinal Ischemia: US-CT findings correlations. Crit Ultrasound J. 2013;5 Suppl 1(Suppl 1):S7. https://doi.org/10.1186/2036-7902-5-S1-S7.

Ripollés T, Simó L, Martínez-Pérez MJ, Pastor MR, Igual A, López A. Sonographic findings in ischemic colitis in 58 patients. AJR Am J Roentgenol. 2005;184(3):777–85. https://doi.org/10.2214/ajr.184.3.01840777.

Chapter 8
Bowel Perforation: Free Air and Free Fluid

Alan Biloslavo, Marina Troian, Diego Mariani, Alessia Malagnino, Antonio La Greca, and Mauro Zago

8.1 Introduction

The presence of free intra-peritoneal air in acutely ill patients represents an important radiological finding that usually indicates a hollow viscus perforation. It can occur for different causes and its detection is critical for diagnosis of potentially life-threatening conditions. In this context, the clinical diagnosis of the site of perforation is not always straightforward as symptoms may be nonspecific. At present, the most common method used to detect free air in the abdomen is plain radiograph of the chest in standing position or plain film of the abdomen in a lateral decubitus view. However, since its reported sensitivity is only 55–85% for detecting small amount of pneumoperitoneum, abdominal computed tomography (CT) is currently considered the gold-standard imaging for recognition, localization, volume, and configuration of free intra-peritoneal air. Nevertheless, it is not a cost-effective option, it determines radiation exposure, and it is potentially harmful in case of use

A. Biloslavo (✉)
Department of General Surgery, ASUGI, Cattinara University Hospital, Trieste, Italy

M. Troian
Cardiothoracic and Vascular Department, ASUGI Cattinara University Hospital, Trieste, Italy

D. Mariani
ASST OVEST Milanese, General Surgery Department, Ospedale di Legnano, Milano, Italy

A. Malagnino · M. Zago
General and Emergency Surgery Unit, General Surgery Department, A. Manzoni Hospital, Lecco, Italy

A. La Greca
Department of Medical and Surgical Sciences, Emergency Surgery Unit, IRCCS Fondazione Policlinico Universitario "A. Gemelli", Catholic University of the Sacred Heart, Rome, Italy

M. Zago et al. (eds.), *Point-of-care US for Acute Abdomen*,
https://doi.org/10.1007/978-3-031-40231-9_8

of contrast means. In addition, patients may be too sick or debilitated to be transported outside the critical ward to undergo a CT scan.

Ultrasonography (US) has emerged as an alternative initial diagnostic tool in patients with acute abdomen, and some researchers have found that US could effectively detect peritoneal-free air. However, reported sensitivity and specificity are ambiguous, and controversies upon its reliability still exist. On the one hand, the obvious shortcoming of US is failure to detect pneumoperitoneum mainly due to the inability to accurately differentiate between intra- and extra-luminal air. On the other hand, US is quick and easy to use, it can be performed bedside, it is radiation-free, and it is cost-effective. Moreover, while both plain radiographs and CT scans provide only still images, US is able to provide real-time in-motion visualization, and it allows the execution of various maneuvers while performing the examination. All these features, together with the possibility of determining not only the presence, but also the cause of pneumoperitoneum, give US a unique and promising lookout for all patients with suspected hollow viscus perforation.

Most important, from a clinical point of view, it should be highlighted that the first intra-abdominal sign of a hollow viscus perforation is free fluid. Starting the US exam with the FAST views, as continuously recommended in this book, could anticipate the confirmation of the diagnosis.

This chapter aims to give the practitioners the fundamentals for performing a US examination in search of pneumoperitoneum, helping them distinguish between intra-luminal and free extra-luminal air through direct and indirect signs, and associated procedures.

8.2 Scanning Technique

The detection of free peritoneal air is difficult even for an experienced sonographer, mainly because extra-luminal air can be mistaken for air *within* the bowel. Other limitations are obesity, subcutaneous emphysema, extensive fecal loading of the colon, lack of patient cooperation, and low quality of some US machines. Therefore, US examination must be meticulous and should not disregard a careful investigation of the patient's history and a scrupulous clinical evaluation whenever possible. Further associated maneuvers, as for instance peritoneal fluid aspiration, may be advised when a high index of suspicion is present despite a lack of direct visualization of free air, or in order to confirm the diagnosis.

The best position to start the US evaluation of the abdomen is the supine decubitus (with a slight chest elevation, if needed). Sagittal and intercostal views, with the probe positioned in the epigastrium and in the right upper quadrant, are the most effective scanning options for free air detection. As in the case of pneumothorax, abdominal free air rises to the highest accessible portion of the peritoneal cavity. Therefore, when performing US in search of pneumoperitoneum, it is worth noting that air usually overlies the liver anteriorly. This explains why it is easier to detect free air between the anterior surface of the left lobe of the liver and the anterior abdominal wall on the midline scan and between the right lobe of the liver and the inner thoracic wall on the right upper quadrant scan.

As for most abdominal pathologies, examination should be started using a curvilinear probe (3.5–5 MHz) to be able to explore the whole abdomen mainly in search of indirect signs of pneumoperitoneum and eventually for a possible etiology. In this context, as explained above, peritoneal effusion is perhaps the most common US finding when hollow viscus perforation is present. However, it is associated with several medical conditions and its detection needs to be contextualized for every single patient. Although the only presence of free fluid is not enough to make a diagnosis of bowel perforation, this additional information may increase the index of a clinical suspicion and may help in the decision-making process.

In the specific search for free gas, it must be noted that linear array probes (7.0–12 MHz) are more sensitive for air detection due to their broader near-field size and the higher resolution. However, most of the times a preliminary scan with only a convex probe will be diagnostic enough to detect free air with no need to shift to a linear one.

On US examination, the gas appears as a bright reflective surface with shadowing that obscures the underlying structures, with either long path reverberation artifacts (like the "A" lines in the lung), in case of large gas collections, or short "ring-down" artifacts, when only bubbles or small amounts of air are present (Fig. 8.1). Extra-luminal air can be found either trapped in an encapsulated collection or free in the peritoneal cavity. In the former case, air can be easily detected at the time of visualization of the collection; in the latter case, air identification may be more challenging.

In physiological conditions, the normal peritoneal stripe is visualized as a single or double echogenic layer deep to the anterior abdominal wall. The presence of peristalsis of the bowel loops is always associated with a normal peritoneal stripe and, in normal conditions, the presence of the so-called gut sliding as well as the detection of the bowel wall allows to rule out pneumoperitoneum.

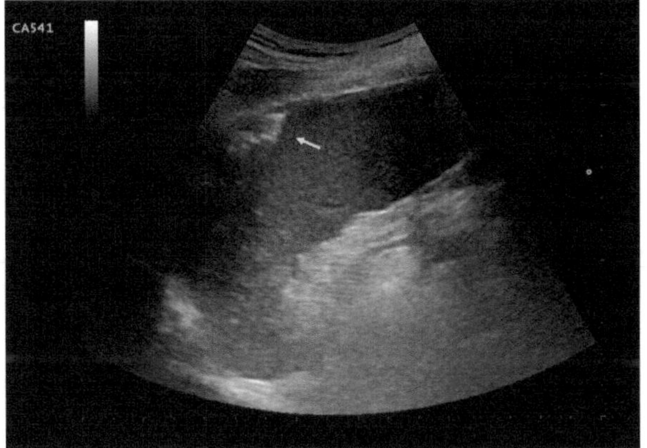

Fig. 8.1 "Ring-down" artifact (*arrow*)

The sonographic appearance of free gas outside the bowel results from scattering of the US waves at the interface between soft tissue and air. Reverberation of the ultrasonic waves between the transducer and the air also results in an increased echogenicity of the peritoneal stripe. This is associated with multiple reflection artifacts and typical "comet tail" appearances. As mentioned above, this physical effect is represented on our machines by echogenic lines or spots with posterior "ring-down" or "comet tails" reverberation artifacts.

The peritoneal stripe thickening sign (Fig. 8.2) was first described by Muradali and colleagues in 1999. Interestingly, this appearance changes when changing the patient's position ("shifting phenomenon"). Conversely, intra-luminal air is always associated with a normal thin peritoneal stripe. Moreover, air inside the bowel moves following the gut peristalsis, and neither gas movements after changing decubitus nor shifting phenomenon can be seen in this case. Thus, once the patient is examined in a supine position, further scans should be obtained both in the left lateral decubitus and eventually in a semi-prone position, consistent with patient's conditions.

US signs of free extra-intestinal gas can be classified into direct and indirect signs. Presence of both direct and indirect signs is associated with a higher sensitivity for pneumoperitoneum.

Direct signs of pneumoperitoneum are:

- Increased echogenicity of peritoneal stripe (peritoneal strip sign, best seen anteriorly to the liver surface).
- Presence of localized gas collection.
- Detection of a step between air in the costophrenic sinus and the abdominal gas reflex.

Indirect signs of pneumoperitoneum are:

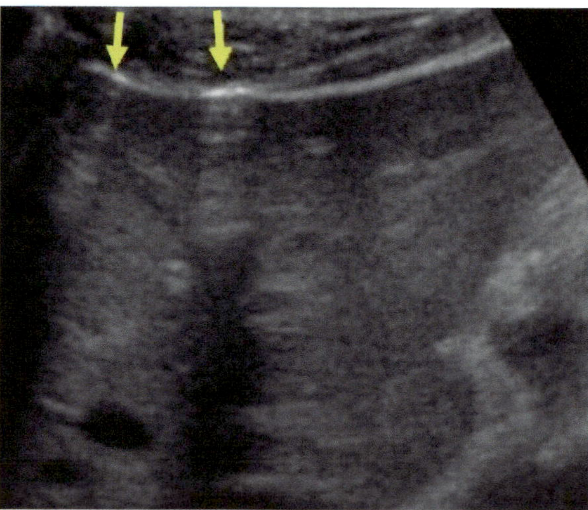

Fig. 8.2 Peritoneal stripe thickening sign (*arrows*)

- Free fluid.
- Thickened bowel loops or thickened gastric wall.
- Ileus (i.e., absence of peristalsis).
- Fluid collections.
- Free air bubbles within a fluid collection.

Additional information aimed at raising the reliability of US investigation can be provided by several specific maneuvers and detection of specific signs. In fact, reverberations are not specific for pneumoperitoneum unless air shifting within the peritoneal cavity is detected by changing decubitus, exerting a gentle pressure with the probe over the belly, or taking advantage from a physiological movement like breathing.

In this context, it is important to remember that during inspiration the lungs move downwards, normally creating the so-called curtain sign at the costophrenic sinus (easily seen in the left upper quadrant, obscuring the spleen at any inspiration). This sign is commonly detected on the right side by scanning the anterior surface of the liver in the right upper quadrant and results from the overlap of the costophrenic recess onto the abdomen, creating a demarcated edge of the lung air which appears like a curtain. Conversely, in the presence of large pneumoperitoneum, an upward movement of the intra-peritoneal air can be observed during exhalation (Fig. 8.3). Moreover, in case of big amounts of extra-luminal air, pneumoperitoneum will overlap the lung at inspiration, thus producing a complete shadowing upon the liver which will then move downward at exhalation, allowing liver visualization again.

Based on the shifting phenomenon concept, in 2004 Karahan and colleagues described the "scissor sign" (Fig. 8.4). This consists in applying and then releasing a slight pressure on the caudal part of a parasagittal or transversally oriented probe,

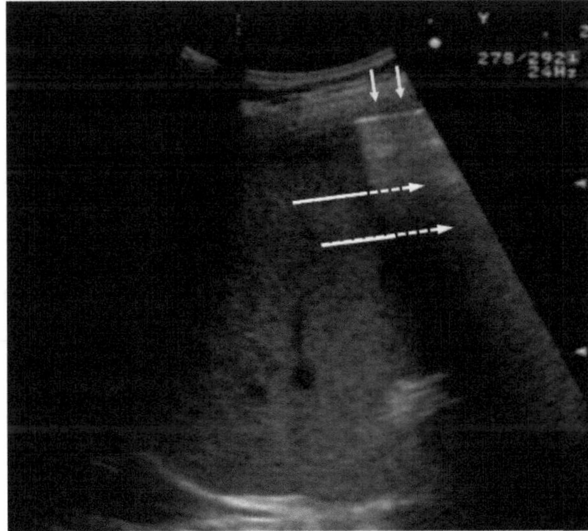

Fig. 8.3 In the presence of pneumoperitoneum, the free air artifacts (*yellow arrows*) are not moving during inspiration and expiration. The liver, "pushed" by the diaphragm during inspiration (*white arrows*), appears to slide under the air artifact. If it would have been within a viscus (i.e., transverse colon), the air artifact would have followed the liver movement

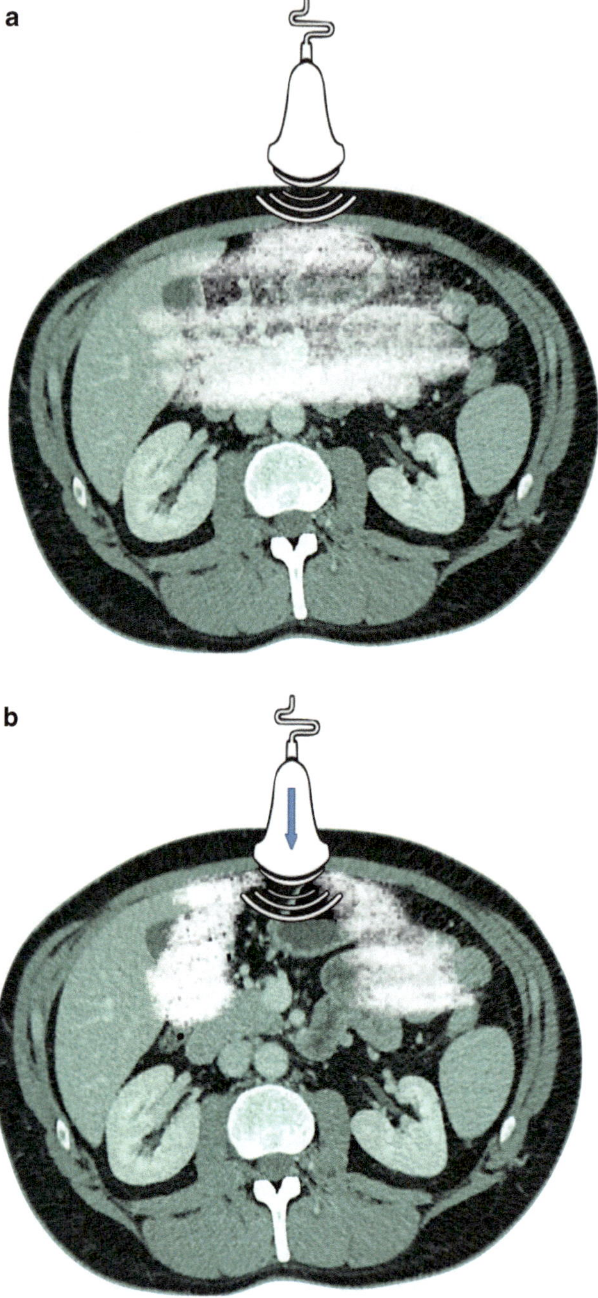

Fig. 8.4 "Scissor sign": by applying and then releasing a slight pressure on the caudal part of a parasagittally/transversally oriented probe placed over a large air artifact (**a**), the gas artifacts become much less prominent during pressure, and could be "scissored" by the probe (**b**)

placed over a large air artifact. Gas artifacts become much less prominent during pressure, and if slightly repeated, the pressure maneuver will entail on the screen the "opening" of the air artifact: half toward the right and half toward the left of the screen, making the probe like a "scissor," cutting the air artifact. Air in a hollow viscus would not be scissored by the probe. In their study, the authors obtained a high diagnostic accuracy, reporting a 94% sensitivity and a 100% specificity, with a PPV of 100% and an NPV of 98%. Notwithstanding, this sign is not routinely easily detected, and it could evocate pain that limits its usefulness.

The shifting phenomenon also represents the basis of what is called the *Zenith sign* (Fig. 8.5). When examining a cooperative patient, with the help of a nurse or a colleague, the probe is first positioned intercostally, on the right midaxillary line, in order to explore the liver and the diaphragm. Once a good US visualization of landmark organs is obtained, the patient is asked to turn on the left side while the

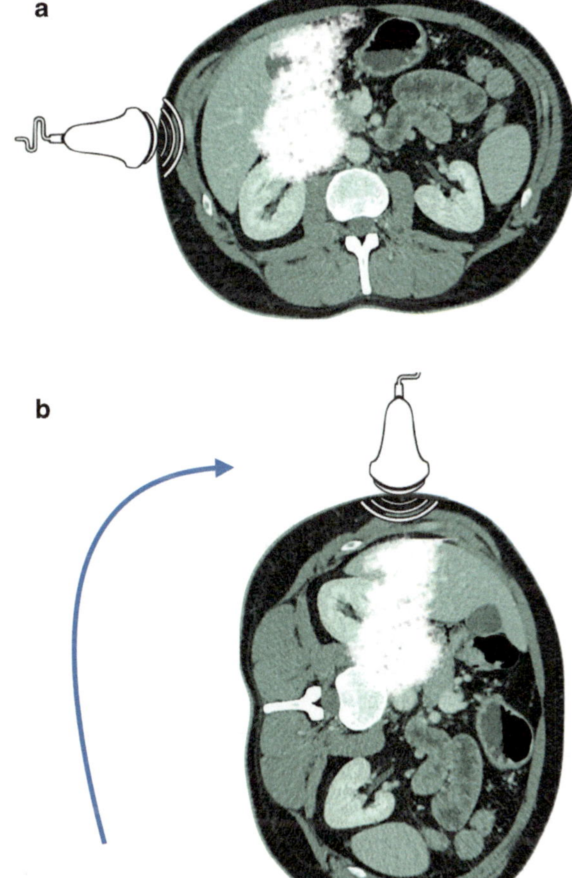

Fig. 8.5 "Zenith sign": moving the patient from the supine to the left lateral decubitus, in case of pneumoperitoneum, free air will initially move upward toward the probe in midaxillary line, producing a shadow effect that obscures the liver (**a**). After reversing the patient's decubitus to the supine position, without moving the probe from the midaxillary line, the air will shift upward again, allowing to see the liver on the monitor again (**b**)

sonographer keeps the probe still in the same position. US is continuously recorded and finally the patient is asked to lay down again on the back, always keeping the probe still. In case of pneumoperitoneum, free air will initially move upward toward the probe producing a shadow effect that obscures the liver in the left lateral decubitus. After reversing the patient's decubitus to the supine position, keeping the probe fixed in the same place, the air will shift upward again, allowing the sonographer to see the liver again on the monitor. The *Zenith sign* is 100% sensitive for the detection of pneumoperitoneum.

Lichtenstein and coworkers tried to combine all the main US signs of pneumoperitoneum in a simple flowchart aimed to help the decision-making process in the US detection of bowel perforation (Fig. 8.6). The scheme is quite simple and easy to use. The first step is recognition of the gut sliding. If present, pneumoperitoneum could reasonably be excluded. If absent, the practitioner should keep looking for the following signs in a consecutive fashion: aerogram and splanchnogram (i.e., when

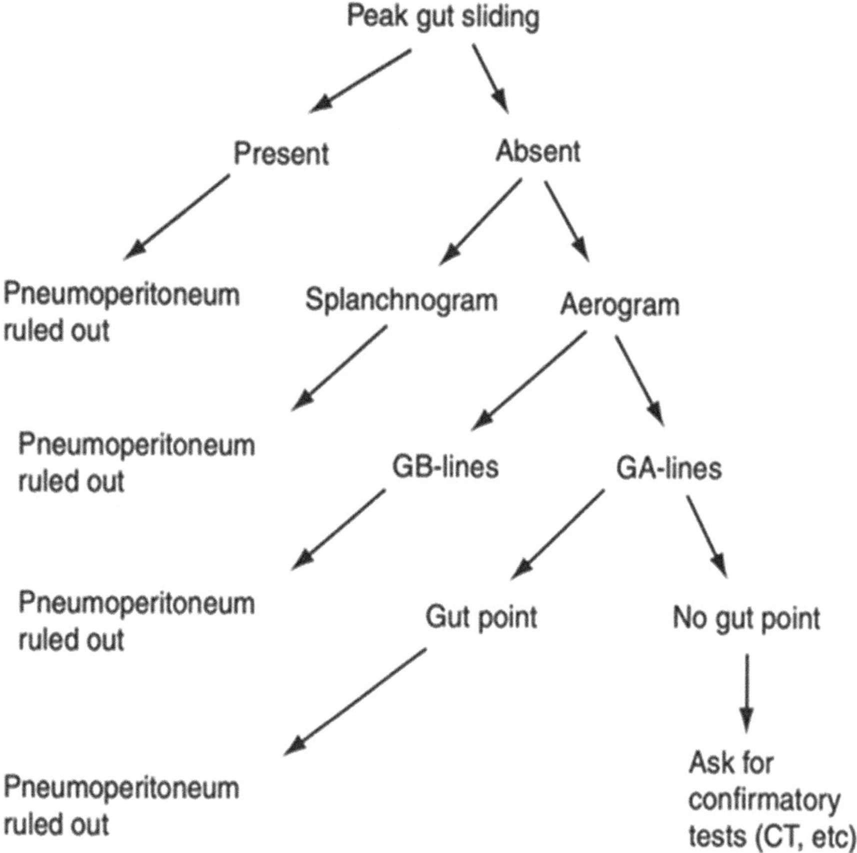

Fig. 8.6 Flowchart proposed by Lichtenstein and colleagues to help the decision-making process in US detection of bowel perforation

an abdominal organ can be seen on US, thus ruling out pneumoperitoneum between the probe and the organ itself), presence of A or B lines, and finally what the authors named *the Gut point* (i.e., the transition zone between normal bowel artifacts, that may normally contain A-lines, and the abnormal A-line pattern without sliding), which is a specific sign with 50% sensitivity. Only in case of undetermined answers, further confirmatory signs and tests are suggested.

Nevertheless, despite the apparent user-friendliness of this flowchart, we believe that the accuracy of US examination aimed at ruling out pneumoperitoneum relies on a meticulous exploration taking into account all of the above-mentioned findings, so as to obtain maximal sensitivity. A methodical approach should be applied proceeding step by step, without forgetting any useful elements. As usual, a careful clinical observation and a high index of suspicion are mandatory to correctly incorporate the imaging findings within the clinical context.

Tips and Tricks

- Start your examination with the patient in a supine position, beginning to scan the upper quadrants. A slight elevation of the chest may be useful
- To differentiate pneumoperitoneum from intra-luminal air, check for the movement of A lines with peristalsis. At the same time, look for enhancement of the peritoneal stripe, as well as reverberation and comet tail artifacts
- The shifting phenomenon (i.e., movement of free air with changes of patient position) is a strong US evidence to support the presence of free air in the abdomen. The Zenith sign is 100% sensitive
- When in doubt, a diagnostic peritoneal aspiration (DPA) of detected free fluid is easy to do and may be helpful in the decision-making process

Red Flags

- *Pitfalls*: patients with peritonitis may present with diminished gut sliding due to antalgic hypopnea. Moreover, gut sliding is hard to detect when the stomach is distended due to its contact with the abdominal wall
- *Warning*: be patient! It is a challenging search but remember US is not the gold standard at pneumoperitoneum detection. Likewise, when taking care of a patient and in doubt if further investigation is needed, US can make the difference in your decision-making process
- *Remember*: free fluid is the first sign of bowel perforation

Appendix: Chapter 7—Test Yourself (Answers in the Appendix at the End of the Book)

Q1—For getting the *Zenith sign*, you need to ask the patient to…

- Turn on the left side.
- Turn on the right side.
- Take a deep breath and hold still.

Q2—The peritoneal stripe thickening sign means…

- Small free fluid collections near the parietal peritoneum.
- A large amount of free air.
- Bubbles of free air "trapped" behind the parietal peritoneum.

Further Reading

Asrani A. Sonographic diagnosis of pneumoperitoneum using the 'enhancement of the peritoneal stripe sign.' A prospective study. Emerg Radiol. 2007;14(1):29–39. https://doi.org/10.1007/s10140-007-0583-3.

Chen SC, Yen ZS, Wang HP, Lin FY, Hsu CY, Chen WJ. Ultrasonography is superior to plain radiography in the diagnosis of pneumoperitoneum. Br J Surg. 2002;89(3):351–4. https://doi.org/10.1046/j.0007-1323.2001.02013.x.

Coppolino F, Gatta G, Di Grezia G, Reginelli A, Iacobellis F, Vallone G, et al. Gastrointestinal perforation: ultrasonographic diagnosis. Crit Ultrasound J. 2013;5 Suppl 1(Suppl 1):S4. https://doi.org/10.1186/2036-7902-5-S1-S4.

Jiang L, Wu J, Feng X. The value of ultrasound in diagnosis of pneumoperitoneum in emergent or critical conditions: A meta-analysis. Hong Kong J Emerg Med. 2019;26(2):111–7. https://doi.org/10.1177/1024907918805668.

Kuzmich S, Burke CJ, Harvey CJ, Kuzmich T, Fascia DT. Sonography of small bowel perforation. AJR Am J Roentgenol. 2013;201(2):W283–91. https://doi.org/10.2214/AJR.12.9882.

Lichtenstein DA. Whole body ultrasound in the critically ill (lung, heart, and venous thrombosis excluded). In: Lung ultrasound in the critically ill. Cham: Springer; 2016. https://doi.org/10.1007/978-3-319-15371-1_34.

Lindelius A, Törngren S, Pettersson H, Adami J. Role of surgeon-performed ultrasound on further management of patients with acute abdominal pain: a randomised controlled clinical trial. Emerg Med J. 2009;26(8):561–6. https://doi.org/10.1136/emj.2008.062067.

Chapter 9
The Thickened Loops: IBD and Surroundings

Giovanni Maconi and Alberta De Monti

9.1 Introduction

Acute abdomen is a clinical condition that requires urgent diagnostic evaluation and treatment. In more than one third of patients, intestinal diseases are the underlying condition and inflammatory bowel diseases (IBDs) are one of these, accounting for up to 3% of total consultations in the emergency department (ED). IBDs (i.e., Crohn's disease, CD, and ulcerative colitis, UC) are chronic inflammatory conditions, characterized by relapsing and remitting episodes of inflammation. The most frequent reasons for urgent consultations are abdominal complications of CD like fistula, abscesses, and obstruction, along with severe flares of the disease, such as bleeding and toxic megacolon, mostly encountered in UC.

The diagnosis of acute abdomen and the detection of its causes are usually easy in patients with known IBD, particularly in those undergoing regular follow-up, but can sometimes be difficult in patients without any history of the disease or complaining atypical symptoms.

Patients with IBD may have systemic symptoms like fever, weakness, and weight loss, and in severe cases they may present with hypotension and tachycardia.

CD is characterized by discontinuous transmural inflammation which may involve any segment of the gastrointestinal tract although approximately 80% of patients have distal or terminal ileum involved. The main symptoms of CD are

G. Maconi (✉)
Gastroenterology Unit, Department of Biomedical and Clinical Sciences, ASST Fatebenefratelli – Sacco University Hospitals, University of Milan, Milan, Italy
e-mail: giovanni.maconi@unimi.it

A. De Monti
Gastroenterology Unit, Department of Oncology, ASST Lecco, "A. Manzoni" Hospital, Lecco, Italy

M. Zago et al. (eds.), *Point-of-care US for Acute Abdomen*,
https://doi.org/10.1007/978-3-031-40231-9_9

crampy abdominal pain, diarrhea (with or without blood), weakness, and weight loss. Symptoms may vary according to the localization of the disease, activity, and complications.

UC is characterized by a continuous inflammation of the mucosal layer of the colon, commonly involving the rectum and possibly spreading proximally up to the cecum and terminal ileum (backwash ileitis) in the more severe conditions. Patients with UC commonly present with bloody diarrhea or blood in the stools, abdominal pain, and urgency.

Despite symptoms being often suggestive of the disease, biochemical tests, endoscopic investigations, and imaging diagnostic techniques are usually performed to confirm the diagnosis, to assess disease activity, and to exclude complications. In recent years, intestinal ultrasound (IUS) has been more frequently used and several international guidelines have recommended it as the first cross-sectional technique to assess patients with clinical suspicion of IBD and to monitor the disease. Systematic reviews and meta-analyses have shown that IUS, and other cross-sectional techniques like Computed Tomography Enterography (CTE) or Magnetic Resonance Enterography (MRE) have similar diagnostic accuracy to detect IBD, particularly CD, and their main abdominal complications. However, US has the advantage of being quick and easy to use, cheap and repeatable.

9.2 Scanning Technique

Intestinal US does not need any specific preparation. However, a moderate filling of the urinary bladder and fasting may be useful.

The assessment of the bowel, even in the suspicion of IBD, usually requires low frequency (3–5 MHz) probes for a general view and to assess deeper parts of the abdomen and pelvis, and high-frequency (5–17 MHz) linear or micro convex probes to better detect the anatomic details of the bowel, superficial parts of the abdomen and the abdominal wall.

Since visualization of the bowel can be hampered by intestinal gas, the gradual compression technique, made with the US probe on the gaseous-filled intestinal loops, usually helps to improve their visualization. The examination should be performed in a systematic way, for example, starting from sigmoid colon to ileocecal region (descending colon, splenic colonic flexure, transverse colon, right colonic flexure, ascending colon). When suspecting an IBD, particular attention must be given to the examination of the ileocecal and recto-sigmoid regions, where CD and UC usually occur, respectively. The well-known reference point for ileocecal region is the right iliac vessels, while the sigmoid colon runs on the left of iliac vessels to the small pelvis.

Anyway, the scan of the whole bowel is recommended in the suspicion of CD because of the well-known segmentary involvement of the disease. Likewise, the assessment of the rectum, through a mildly filled bladder in hypogastrium, pushing hard to reach the correct depth, should be used in the suspicion of UC.

In these areas, the following sonographic features of the intestinal wall must be described: wall-thickness, stratification, echogenicity, length of affected segment, luminal width, vascularization, and peristalsis. Associated findings in adjacent mesenteric tissue and lymph nodes are also important findings to report.

9.2.1 Crohn's Disease (CD)

CD may be detected and suspected by IUS in the presence of the following features: increased bowel wall thickening >3 mm, possible focal or extensive disruption of the normal wall stratification, and increased bowel wall vascularization.

9.2.1.1 Thickening of Bowel Wall

This is the most important and reproducible sonographic parameter to detect IBD. The wall thickening should be measured in both longitudinal and transversal sections, from the inner interface between hyperechoic (interface) and hypoechoic (mucosa) layers to the outer interface between hypoechoic (muscularis) and hyperechoic (serosa) layers (Fig. 9.1).

The measurement of the maximum bowel wall thickness should be taken where the bowel damage is more representative, possibly both on the anterior and posterior walls, and on two different quadrants of a transversal scan of the loop. The average

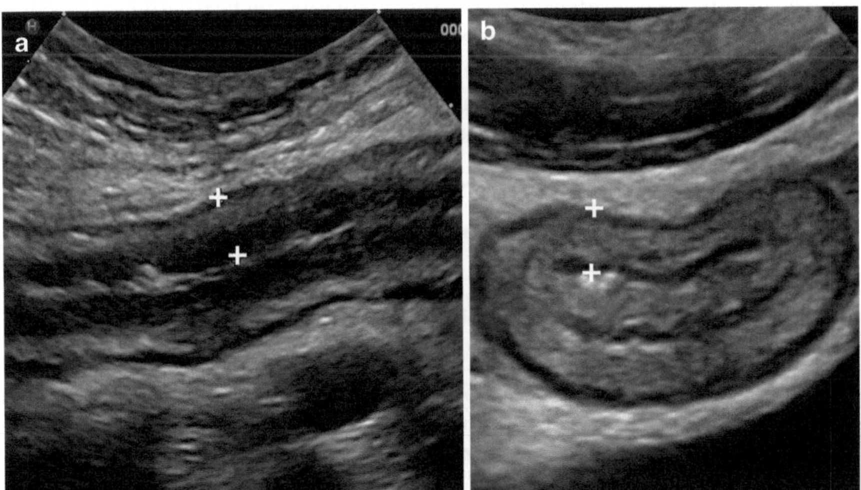

Fig. 9.1 Thickening of the bowel wall measured (+) both in longitudinal (*a*, left panel) and transversal (*b*, right panel) sections, from the inner interface between hyperechoic (interface) and hypoechoic (mucosa) layers to the outer interface between hypoechoic (muscularis) and hyperechoic (serosa) layers

of the measurements of the thickening (along with the range) should be reported and considered pathological and suspicious for IBD when >3 mm. This specific cut-off, according to literature meta-analyses, gives a sensitivity and specificity in the detection of IBD of 89% and 96%, respectively.

In patients with acute abdomen, IBDs are usually associated with a more severe bowel damage and/or abdominal complications and are therefore easier to detect by IUS. The thickening should be assessed, considering its length, together with the compressibility, peristalsis, presence or disruption of the normal stratification, and vascularization.

9.2.1.2 Echo Pattern

The thickened bowel walls may be characterized by a preserved stratification or by a focal or extensive disruption of stratification. The loss of stratification correlates with the presence of deep ulcers and neoangiogenesis, thus implying a more severe disease activity (Fig. 9.2). Unfortunately, the assessment of echo pattern, despite relevant for evaluating disease activity, is reported with limited reproducibility mainly due to frequency of the probe, operator experience and likely the kind of the sonographic machine.

9.2.1.3 Vascularity

This parameter reflects neoangiogenesis, and it is therefore more closely and directly correlated with disease activity. Bowel wall vascularity can be determined by color Doppler US or contrast enhanced ultrasound (CEUS) and evaluated by using semi-quantitative or quantitative indexes. Like the evaluation of echo pattern, the assessment of vascularity is subjected to limited reproducibility and affected by operator experience as well as by the type and setting of the machine.

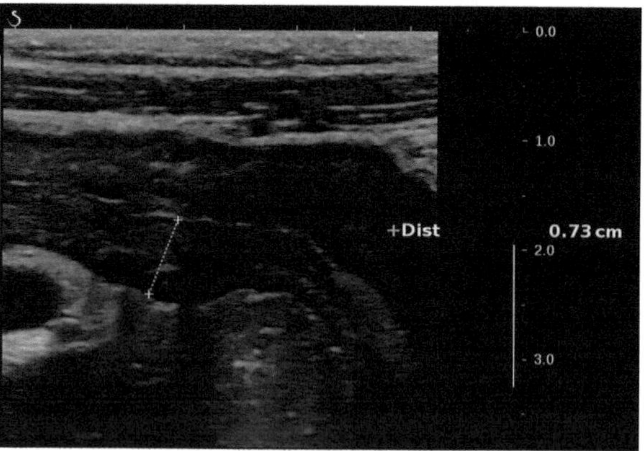

Fig. 9.2 Thickening bowel wall characterized by an extensive disruption of stratification

9.2.1.4 Extraintestinal Features

The evaluation of the bowel in patients with suspected or known IBD should always include the assessment of extraintestinal findings, in particular mesenteric lymph nodes and mesenteric fat.

Enlarged mesenteric lymph nodes should be evaluated and reported, with specific interest regarding their shape and site. Oval or elongated shape is more typical for reactive nodes due to inflammatory or infectious diseases, while round shape is more suspicious for neoplastic diseases. The size to discriminate normal from pathological lymph nodes, whether reactive or neoplastic, is still controversial. Generally, a pathological lymph node is reported to have a lesser diameter >4 mm in adults and >8 mm in children, and these measures are usually considered also for CD patients. In CD, they are usually found at the mesenteric root and mainly in the right lower and upper left quadrants. The presence of lymph nodes is usually correlated with young age, early disease, and abdominal septic complications like fistulas and abscesses (Fig. 9.3).

Mesenteric fat hypertrophy appears as bright hyperechoic tissue surrounding inflamed bowel loops and thickened bowel wall. It is associated with transmural inflammation, clinical and biochemical disease activity (Fig. 9.4).

9.2.2 Ulcerative Colitis (UC)

The role of IUS in UC is less defined than in CD, likely because inflammatory lesions in UC are confined to the colon and often the rectum, which is difficult to image by US, and also because of milder pathological involvement of the bowel wall, confined to the inner mucosal layer. Colonoscopy is therefore the diagnostic method of choice and the reference standard in UC.

However, IUS is an accurate tool to define the extension of the disease and its activity. The more typical sonographic features are a *moderate thickening of the*

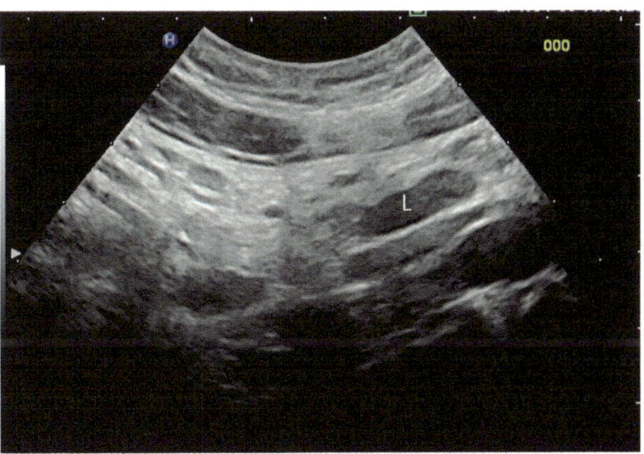

Fig. 9.3 Enlarged reactive mesenteric lymph node found at the mesenteric root in a patient with Crohn's disease

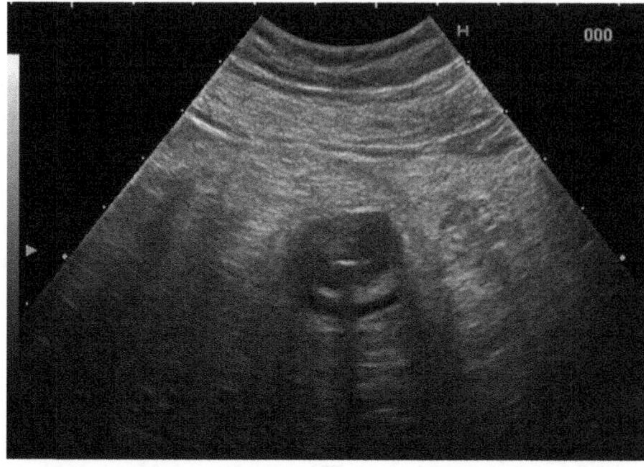

Fig. 9.4 Mesenteric fat hypertrophy appearing as bright hyperechoic tissue surrounding inflamed bowel loops with thickened bowel wall

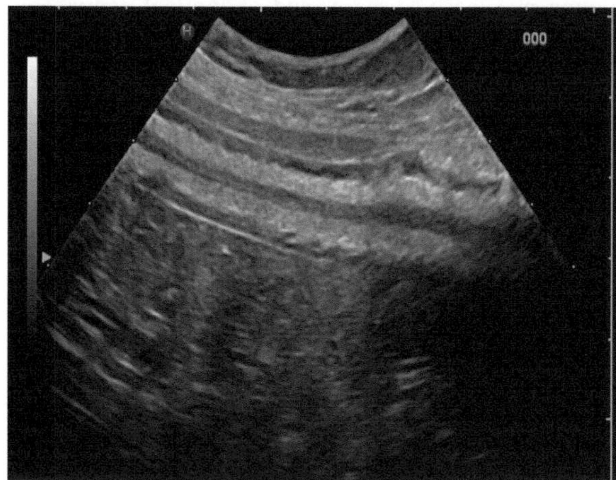

Fig. 9.5 Thickening of the colonic wall with preserved wall stratification, regular margins, and loss of haustration

*mucosa and submucosa laye*r (usually >3 mm and <9 mm), *usually with preserved stratification*—except for severely active UC, where focal or extensive disruption of wall stratification may be observed due to the presence of deep ulcers. *Loss of haustration* is another common finding (Fig. 9.5).

Regarding the limitation of rectal assessment in UC, this can be overcome by using trans-perineal US, which—combined with trans-abdominal US—visualizes the colon and rectum and can be very useful to monitor disease activity after therapy.

9.3 Clinical Meanings of Abnormal Findings

9.3.1 CD Complications

The new onset of disease, clinical recurrences, and abdominal complications are frequent reasons for ED consultation. Specifically, abdominal complications of CD are the most frequent reason for ED consultation and the main indication for surgery in patients with IBDs. In fact, the 10-year risk of surgery for CD patients is nearly 50%.

9.3.1.1 Stenosis and Occlusion

These are the most frequent intestinal complications of CD and cause of surgery in 70–90% of cases. Strictures may be due to either thickened bowel wall with progressive narrowing of the lumen or adhesions. Both conditions can lead to mechanical (complete or incomplete) bowel obstruction.

Small bowel occlusion is characterized by an abnormal dilatation (> 2.5–3 cm) with static, swirling contents (Fig. 9.6). In CD, this can be appreciable just before a stricture (*pre-stenotic dilatation*), characterized by a thickened bowel wall, with narrowed lumen (diameter < 1 cm), and a usually fixed segment of the bowel (Fig. 9.7). In chronic occlusion, the real-time evaluation usually detects a slow peristalsis, as opposed to the acute mechanical occlusion where a dysfunctional hyperperistalsis is more frequently present. Colonic obstruction is usually seen as an abrupt transition from a normal to a pathological dilatation (>4–5 cm) with liquid (right colon) or solid content (left colon).

The sensitivity of IUS in detecting the stenosis is approximately 80–85%. However, it may be improved by using small intestinal contrast agents, namely PEG

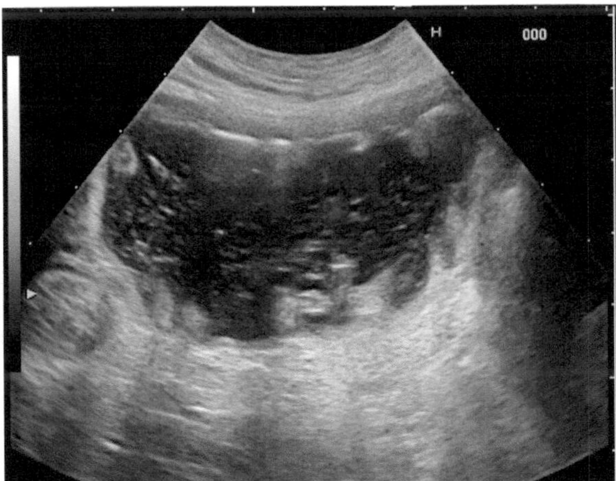

Fig. 9.6 Small bowel obstruction characterized by abnormal dilatation (>2.5–3 cm) of bowel loops with liquid content

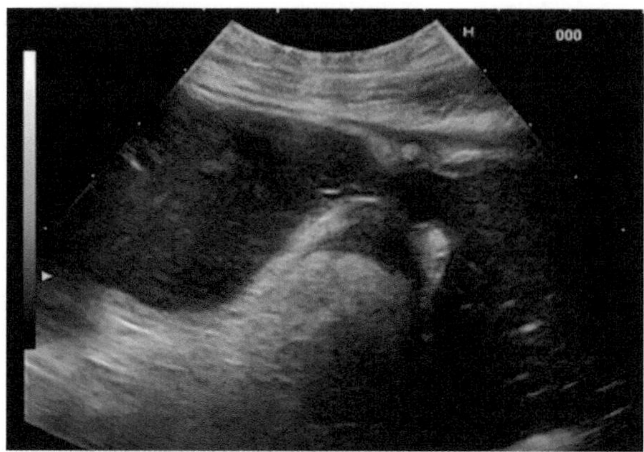

Fig. 9.7 Longitudinal scan of a short, small bowel stricture characterized by thickened bowel walls, narrowing of the lumen, and bowel dilatation, in patients with small bowel obstruction and multiple bowel strictures

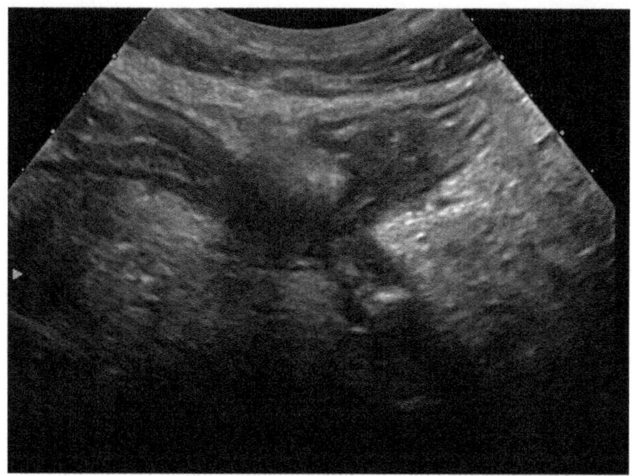

Fig. 9.8 Intestinal fistulas are pathological connections between two epithelialized structures, which appear at IUS as hypoechoic tracts between intestinal loops or between loops and other organs

solution in amount of 500–800 mL, which should be drunk 30 min prior to the exam. The use of PEG (Small Intestinal Contrast Ultrasound, SICUS) can increase the sensitivity in detecting strictures of 10–20%.

9.3.1.2 Fistulas and Perforation

Intestinal fistulas are pathological connections between two epithelialized structures, which appear on IUS as hypoechoic tracts between intestinal loops or between loops and other organs, like the urinary bladder or the skin (Fig. 9.8). Fistulas can present internal hyperechoic content (i.e., air, debris, or intestinal content), but can also appear as an empty and virtual lumen. The accuracy of IUS in detecting fistulas shows a sensitivity of 74% and a specificity of 95%.

Perforations or microperforation could be considered as a sort of early internal fistulas as they are consequences of deep fissures in the wall of the loop involved. Free perforation can be suspected in the presence of free fluid or intraperitoneal air, but it is more frequent to identify a focal buffered perforation appearing as a small collection of air or fluid near a pathological loop. The site of microperforation may be seen as a small alteration of the outer serosal surface, which is otherwise normally smooth.

9.3.1.3 Abscess and Phlegmons

Abscesses are fluid collections which usually appear as hypo- or anechoic areas surrounded by hypertrophic and bright mesenteric fat, sometimes with small bright hyperechoic spots suggesting presence of air inside (Fig. 9.9). Phlegmons are less organized inflammatory hypoechoic masses with no clear wall or fluid content, often indistinguishable from abscesses, unless intravenous (IV) contrast agents are used. Despite its limitations and even without the use of IV contrast, the sensitivity and specificity of IUS for identification of these lesions is still 93% and 84%, respectively.

9.3.2 UC Complications

The main reasons for ED consultation in UC patients are the new onset of the disease and its flare, particularly if the disease presents acutely or associated with an intestinal complication.

9.3.2.1 Severe Disease Activity

In this context, IUS is usually performed to confirm the severity and assess the extent of the disease.

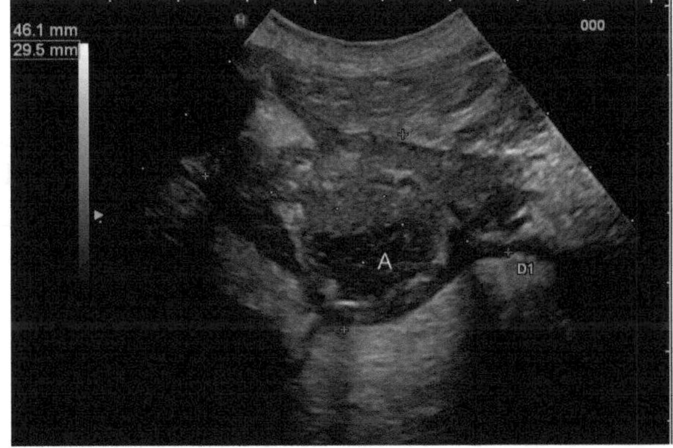

Fig. 9.9 Abdominal mesenteric abscess (*A*), appearing as hypo- or anechoic area, surrounded by hypertrophic and bright mesenteric fat, with small bright hyperechoic spots suggesting the presence of air inside

9.3.2.2 Toxic Megacolon

This is a severe complication of UC characterized by non-obstructive colonic dilatation associated with systemic toxicity. The presence of toxic megacolon should be suspected when there is a strong decrease of the thickening in the colonic wall (<2 mm) with concurrent dilatation of the colon (>6 cm). In these situations, it is also common to find free fluid and dilatation of ileal loops. Plain abdominal X-ray and/or abdominal CT scan are mandatory radiological examinations to accurately assess the extent of this complication anyway.

9.4 Differential Diagnosis of IBDs

The sonographic differential diagnosis between IBDs and other inflammatory conditions (i.e., ischemic colitis and infectious enterocolitis) can sometimes be very difficult or nearly impossible, especially in people of advanced age.

Infectious enterocolitis may have ultrasound features similar to those of UC and CD. Generally, enteritis caused by Salmonella, Yersinia, and Campylobacter often involve the right colon and the cecum as well as the terminal ileum, causing modest or slight thickening of the bowel walls, which however maintain regular stratification, elasticity, and peristalsis. Infectious enteritis are often associated with lymphadenomegaly (in particular, Yersinia enterocolitica enteritis and salmonellosis), where enlarged lymph nodes are sometimes arranged in a "chain of rosary" fashion along the right iliac artery. *Intestinal tuberculosis* involves right colon and ileum, with a parietal involvement like that of CD, and sometimes it is characterized by marked bowel wall thickening with hypoechoic echo pattern, irregular margins, and possible coexistence of fistulas.

Pseudomembranous colitis is usually suspected after a recent antibiotic treatment, based on clinical history and acute onset, in the absence of hematochezia. On IUS, the colic walls will appear markedly thickened, although elastic and folded like an "accordion," with inhomogeneous echogenic material within the lumen (Fig. 9.10).

In case of *ischemic colitis*, the chronic ischemic involvement of the walls sometimes has endoscopic, histological, and thus also sonographic characteristics very similar to those of chronic inflammatory colitis, such as to make this condition very difficult to distinguish from inflammatory colitis. Therefore, the clinical context and the assessment of splanchnic circulation, in particular by means of Doppler evaluation of the superior and inferior mesenteric arteries, may help in the differential diagnosis.

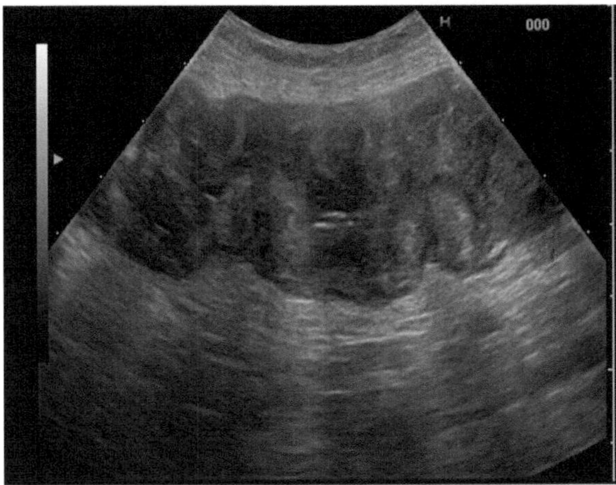

Fig. 9.10 Pseudomembranous colitis appearing as markedly thickened colonic walls, with elastic and preserved folds and haustrations arranged as an "accordion" (accordion sign), with inhomogeneous echogenic material within the lumen

Tips and Tricks

- Gradual compression to improve visualization
- Correct assessment of the wall: thickening, stratification, vascularization
- Use of contrast agents: oral media improve detection of strictures, intravenous media discriminate phlegmons and abscesses

Remember!

- *Measures*
  - Pathological thickening: >3 mm
  - Pathological lymph nodes: >4 mm in adults, >8 mm in children
  - Pathological pre-stenotic dilatation: >2.5–3 cm in the small bowel, >4–5 cm in the colon
- *CD complications*
  - *Stenosis*: thickened, fixed segment with narrowed lumen associated with pre-stenotic dilatation with static, swirling contents
  - *Fistulas*: hypoechoic tracts with internal echoic spots
  - *Abscess*: hypoechoic fluid collections with bright echogenicity

Appendix: Chapter 8—Test Yourself (Answers in the Appendix at the End of the Book)

Q1—Pre-stenotic dilation in Crohn's disease is defined as…?

- >25–30 mm
- >40 mm
- >50 mm

Q2—Pathological thickening of a bowel wall is…

- >4 mm
- >3 mm

Further Reading

Dietrich CF, Hollerweger A, Dirks K, Higginson A, Serra C, Calabrese E, et al. EFSUMB gastrointestinal ultrasound (GIUS) task force group: celiac sprue and other rare gastrointestinal diseases ultrasound features. Med Ultrason. 2019;21(3):299–315. https://doi.org/10.11152/mu-2162.

Frolkis AD, Dykeman J, Negrón ME, Debruyn J, Jette N, Fiest KM, et al. Risk of surgery for inflammatory bowel diseases has decreased over time: a systematic review and meta-analysis of population-based studies. Gastroenterology. 2013;145(5):996–1006. https://doi.org/10.1053/j.gastro.2013.07.041.

Gottlieb M, Peksa GD, Pandurangadu AV, Nakitende D, Takhar S, Seethala RR. Utilization of ultrasound for the evaluation of small bowel obstruction: A systematic review and meta-analysis. Am J Emerg Med. 2018;36(2):234–42. https://doi.org/10.1016/j.ajem.2017.07.085.

Hollerweger A, Maconi G, Ripolles T, Nylund K, Higginson A, Serra C, et al. Gastrointestinal ultrasound (GIUS) in intestinal emergencies - an EFSUMB position paper. Ultraschall Med. 2020;41(6):646–57; English. https://doi.org/10.1055/a-1147-1295.

Laméris W, van Randen A, van Es HW, van Heesewijk JP, van Ramshorst B, Bouma WH, et al. Imaging strategies for detection of urgent conditions in patients with acute abdominal pain: diagnostic accuracy study. BMJ. 2009;338:b2431. https://doi.org/10.1136/bmj.b2431.

Lichtenstein GR, Loftus EV, Isaacs KL, Regueiro MD, Gerson LB, Sands BE. ACG clinical guideline: management of Crohn's disease in adults. Am J Gastroenterol. 2018;113(4):481–517. https://doi.org/10.1038/ajg.2018.27; Epub 2018 Mar 27. Erratum in: Am J Gastroenterol. 2018 Jul;113(7):1101.

Lu C, Merrill C, Medellin A, Novak K, Wilson SR. Bowel Ultrasound State of the Art: Grayscale and Doppler Ultrasound, Contrast Enhancement, and Elastography in Crohn Disease. J Ultrasound Med. 2019 Feb;38(2):271–88. https://doi.org/10.1002/jum.14920.

Maaser C, Sturm A, Vavricka SR, Kucharzik T, Fiorino G, Annese V, et al. ECCO-ESGAR guideline for diagnostic assessment in IBD part 1: initial diagnosis, monitoring of known IBD, detection of complications. J Crohns Colitis. 2019;13(2):144–64. https://doi.org/10.1093/ecco-jcc/jjy113.

Maconi G, Radice E, Greco S, Bianchi PG. Bowel ultrasound in Crohn's disease. Best Pract Res Clin Gastroenterol. 2006;20(1):93–112. https://doi.org/10.1016/j.bpg.2005.09.001.

Maconi G, Greco S, Duca P, Ardizzone S, Massari A, Cassinotti A, et al. Prevalence and clinical significance of sonographic evidence of mesenteric fat alterations in Crohn's disease. Inflamm Bowel Dis. 2008;14(11):1555–61. https://doi.org/10.1002/ibd.20515.

Maconi G, Nylund K, Ripolles T, Calabrese E, Dirks K, Dietrich CF, et al. EFSUMB recommendations and clinical guidelines for intestinal ultrasound (GIUS) in inflammatory bowel diseases. Ultraschall Med. 2018;39(3):304–17; English. https://doi.org/10.1055/s-0043-125329.

Magro F, Gionchetti P, Eliakim R, Ardizzone S, Armuzzi A, Barreiro-de Acosta M, et al. Third European evidence-based consensus on diagnosis and management of ulcerative colitis. Part 1: definitions, diagnosis, extra-intestinal manifestations, pregnancy, cancer surveillance, surgery, and ileo-anal pouch disorders. J Crohns Colitis. 2017;11(6):649–70. https://doi.org/10.1093/ecco-jcc/jjx008; Erratum in: J Crohns Colitis. 2022 Aug 16.

Murata A, Okamoto K, Mayumi T, Maramatsu K, Matsuda S. Age-related differences in outcomes and etiologies of acute abdominal pain based on a national administrative database. Tohoku J Exp Med. 2014;233(1):9–15. https://doi.org/10.1620/tjem.233.9.

Nylund K, Maconi G, Hollerweger A, Ripolles T, Pallotta N, Higginson A, et al. EFSUMB recommendations and guidelines for gastrointestinal ultrasound. Ultraschall Med. 2017;38(3):e1–e15; English. https://doi.org/10.1055/s-0042-115853.

Panés J, Bouzas R, Chaparro M, García-Sánchez V, Gisbert JP, Martínez de Guereñu B, et al. Systematic review: the use of ultrasonography, computed tomography and magnetic resonance imaging for the diagnosis, assessment of activity and abdominal complications of Crohn's disease. Aliment Pharmacol Ther. 2011;34(2):125–45. https://doi.org/10.1111/j.1365-2036.2011.04710.x.

Sagami S, Kobayashi T, Aihara K, Umeda M, Morikubo H, Matsubayashi M, et al. Transperineal ultrasound predicts endoscopic and histological healing in ulcerative colitis. Aliment Pharmacol Ther. 2020;51(12):1373–83. https://doi.org/10.1111/apt.15767.

Silverberg MS, Satsangi J, Ahmad T, Arnott ID, Bernstein CN, Brant SR, et al. Toward an integrated clinical, molecular and serological classification of inflammatory bowel disease: report of a Working Party of the 2005 Montreal World Congress of Gastroenterology. Can J Gastroenterol. 2005;19 Suppl A:5A–36A. https://doi.org/10.1155/2005/269076.

Strobel D, Goertz RS, Bernatik T. Diagnostics in inflammatory bowel disease: ultrasound. World J Gastroenterol. 2011;17(27):3192–7. https://doi.org/10.3748/wjg.v17.i27.3192.

Chapter 10
CEUS in Visceral Emergencies

Diego Mariani, Alan Biloslavo, Giovanni Maconi, Matteo Marconi, Marina Troian, and Mauro Zago

10.1 Introduction

The basic physical principle for contrast-enhanced US (CEUS) relies on the unique interaction between high-frequency sound waves and microbubbles. Specifically, US contrast media are made up of tiny gas bubbles that present a higher acoustic impedance than that of the encircling blood, thus determining linear reflections as it occurs for static soft tissue. However, since the microbubbles are smaller than the wavelength of the US beam, they oscillate following the course of the sound wave, becoming rhythmically larger and smaller and resulting in a non-linear backscatter. As the acoustic pressure increases, the microbubbles oscillate more strongly, until they expand beyond their limit and burst ("cavitation effect"). The combination of signals generated by the oscillation and destruction of microbubbles determines a

D. Mariani (✉)
ASST OVEST Milanese, General Surgery Department, Ospedale di Legnano, Milano, Italy

A. Biloslavo
Department of General Surgery, ASUGI, Cattinara University Hospital, Trieste, Italy

G. Maconi
Gastroenterology Unit, Department of Biomedical and Clinical Sciences, ASST Fatebenefratelli – Sacco University Hospitals, University of Milan, Milan, Italy

M. Marconi
General Surgery Department, ASST Ovest Milanese, "G. Fornaroli" Hospital, Milan, Italy

M. Troian
Cardiothoracic and Vascular Department, ASUGI Cattinara University Hospital, Trieste, Italy

M. Zago
General and Emergency Surgery Unit, General Surgery Department, A. Manzoni Hospital, Lecco, Italy

M. Zago et al. (eds.), *Point-of-care US for Acute Abdomen*,
https://doi.org/10.1007/978-3-031-40231-9_10

marked amplification of the blood flow, creating the CEUS images. This technology requires the use of dedicated software to improve contrast resolution and suppress stationary signals from the surrounding tissues. A split screen allows for simultaneous view of baseline greyscale and contrast-enhanced images.

US contrast media are intravascular agents that do not pass through the endothelial wall and technological research has focused on the optimal development of an inert inner gas bubble surrounded by a stabilizing outer shell. Ideally, the bubbles should have an adequate size to pass the blood–air barrier in the lungs. Currently, the diameter of commercially available US contrast agents varies between 1 μm and 7 μm. Too small bubbles are unstable and do not resist long enough in the bloodstream, whereas bubbles larger than 10 μm creates a temporary obstacle in the capillary circulation. Moreover, the gas-filled microbubbles must have a low solubility in blood plasma, and they are coated with a protective outer shell of various composition (i.e., proteins, lipids, polymers), that does not modify the acoustic beam and maintains its characteristics through tissue metabolism to persist long enough into the bloodstream.

Generally, the contrast agent is administered intravenously. The arterial phase begins 10–20 s after the injection and lasts up to 30–40 s thereafter. Over time, the concentration of the microbubbles in the capillary beds decreases, and it is excreted through the air breath. The late venous distribution is specific for each tissue and changes continuously during the scanning, allowing for real-time visualization of parenchymal perfusion.

Nowadays, US contrast agents are categorized according to the type of gas within the microbubble shell. First-generation US contrast media were characterized by air-filled microbubbles with high mechanical index and a limited lifetime, rapidly dissolving when exposed to the acoustic pressure of the US beam. Second-generation US contrast media present a gaseous content with lower plasma solubility and a more stable outer shell. Working with a lower mechanical index, they last longer in the bloodstream, producing non-linear harmonic frequencies that are detected by the US machine, creating the contrast-enhanced image. Table 10.1 summarizes some of the most frequently used contrast media.

10.2 Scanning Technique

Although visceral US was not considered feasible until the 1970s, this technique has since long demonstrated its ability in the evaluation of intestinal loops. In this context, the US examination usually begins with low-frequency convex probes (i.e., 3.5–5.0 MHz), which allow for a gross assessment of the gastrointestinal tract. Then, high-frequency linear probes (5.0–10.0 MHz) can be used to obtain a more detailed high-resolution image. However, this could be limited by the thickness of the abdominal wall, possibly preventing an adequate visceral scanning.

Remember that to perform CEUS, contrast-specific software is required to be installed on the ultrasound device. This is generally available on high-end

Table 10.1 Types of commercially available US contrast media

First-generation US contrast media	
Levovist® (Schering AG, Berlin, Germany)	
Year of production	1996
Gas used	Air
Protective shell	Galactose (99.9%), palmitic acid (0.1%)
Field of application	Cardiology, internal medicine. Designed to amplify the Doppler US signal, it was progressively employed in the characterization of liver lesions, in transcranial Doppler examinations, and in the study of pediatric vesico-ureteral reflux
Contraindications	Galactosemia. No data for pregnancy and breast-feeding status
Side-effects	Headache, nausea, changes in arterial blood pressure, changes in heart rate, skin rash. Use with caution in patients with severe cardiac insufficiency
Second-generation US contrast media	
Optison® (GE Healthcare, Princeton, NJ, USA)	
Year of production	1997
Gas used	Perflutren
Protective shell	Human serum albumin
Field of application	Cardiovascular imaging, focal liver lesions evaluation
Contraindications	Congestive heart failure, right-to-left cardiac shunts, severe respiratory failure, hypersensitivity to blood products or albumin
Side-effects	Headache, nausea/vomiting, warm sensation or flushing, dizziness
SonoVue® (Bracco, Milano, Italy)	
Year of production	2001
Gas used	Sulfur hexafluoride
Protective shell	Phospholipids
Field of application	Echocardiography, Doppler tests for large blood vessels (e.g., head, liver, thyroid, kidney, soft tissue neoplasms, lymph nodes), pediatric vesico-ureteral reflux
Contraindications	Acute myocardial infarction, heart failure, right-to-left cardiac shunts, severe pulmonary hypertension, adult respiratory distress syndrome
Side-effects	Headache, nausea, injection site pain, skin rash, abdominal/chest pain, vasodilation, hyperglycemia, dizziness, blurred vision, alteration of taste
Luminity® (Bristol-Myers Squibb, Brussels, Belgium)	
Year of production	2006
Gas used	Octafluoropropane
Protective shell	Phospholipids
Field of application	Cardiology
Contraindications	Hypersensitivity, acute myocardial infarction, severe respiratory distress syndrome

(continued)

Table 10.1 (continued)

Side-effects	Headache, skin rash, back pain, abdominal pain, dizziness, paresthesia, alteration in cardiac rhythm, palpitation, hypotension, nausea/vomiting
Sonazoid® (GE Healthcare, Waukesha, WI, USA)	
Year of production	2007
Gas used	Perfluorobutane
Protective shell	Hydrogenated egg phosphatidyl serine embedded in an amorphous sucrose structure
Field of application	Focal liver lesions evaluation, focal breast lesions evaluation
Contraindications	Hypersensitivity and history of allergy to eggs or eggs products, patients with right-left arteriovenous cardiac or pulmonary lungs, serious pulmonary and/or coronary arterial disease
Side-effects	Headache, diarrhea, nausea, vomiting, abdominal pain, transient altered taste, fever

equipment. However, keep in mind that the software may not be installed on every probe: generally, convex probes are the ones supported.

When the examination site has been identified, both sagittal and transverse scans are required. Under normal circumstances, the bowel is compressible and presents five sonographic layers resulting from a combination of interface echoes of the different histological sections.

When using a contrast agent, it is of paramount importance to know its characteristics, posology, and method of administration. In Europe, the most used contrast agent is SonoVue®, containing sulfur hexafluoride. It is administered by intravenous injection of 2.0–2.4 mL bolus, followed by a flush of 5.0–10.0 mL of 0.9% sodium chloride. Generally, two separate boluses are administered, in order to accurately evaluate the organs both on the right side and on the left side of the abdomen. Visualization of both visceral walls and parenchymal tissues will differ according to the time elapsed since infusion and circulation refill specific for each organ.

10.3 CEUS Applications in Visceral US

10.3.1 Inflammatory Bowel Disease

The clinical manifestations of inflammatory bowel diseases (IBDs) can vary greatly in terms of signs, symptoms, age of onset, and natural history. Generally, the inflammatory process involves the whole intestinal wall and can extend to the adjacent mesentery and surrounding lymphatic tissue. Although several laboratory parameters have been proposed to identify the state of activity of the inflammatory process, none has been found to be totally reliable.

Recently, visceral US has proved to be an important, consistent, non-invasive tool in the diagnosis and follow-up of patients with IBDs (see Chap. 8 for more detailed information). Specifically, intestinal hyperemia is an unequivocal sign of active disease and can be clearly highlighted during standard examination with Doppler US. Unfortunately, this type of investigation is not always easy to perform because of bowel movements preventing appropriate Doppler assessment. Hence, the evaluation can be improved by using contrast agents, as CEUS is not affected by peristalsis, and it allows a clear identification of blood flows. In patients with active disease, the contrast medium will be taken up by the bowel, confirming the state of acute inflammation. In this context, Di Sabatino and colleagues demonstrated in 2002 that intravenous administration of microbubble US contrast agent (i.e., Levovist®) markedly enhanced Doppler signal intensity, increasing sensitivity for Crohn's disease from 71% to 97%.

The use of contrast media seems to correlate well also in the subclinical phase of the disease, allowing for early identification of inflammatory processes as well as adequate evaluation of follow-up and response to therapy. For these reasons, the use of CEUS in patients with IBD represents an effective tool in monitoring the evolution of a constantly changing pathology and may help in the decision-making process of the most appropriate treatment.

10.3.2 Intestinal Ischemia

Few studies evaluated the role of CEUS in the assessment of intestinal ischemia. The most significant papers were published in 2005 and in 2007 by two Japanese groups of gastroenterologists. According to their prospective evaluation, the use of US contrast media is characterized by a good accuracy in the early diagnosis of visceral ischemia. In both studies, CEUS was found to have a sensitivity of nearly 90% and a specificity close to 100% compared to intraoperative findings.

10.3.3 Acute Appendicitis and Diverticulitis

Under normal circumstances, the appendix results as a compressible, non-painful, blind-ending, tubular structure with a diameter of less than 6 mm on conventional US. The vascular pattern on Doppler examination is seldom evident, as the blood flow is usually too slow to be detected. In case of acute inflammation, the diameter becomes thicker, and the blood flow increases, both in representation and in speed.

In this context, conventional US has a sensitivity of 89% and a specificity of 95% for the diagnosis of acute appendicitis. By utilizing US contrast agents, the sensitivity has been shown to increase up to 100% as the modifications in blood flow are more easily detected. However, CEUS has hardly any clinical significance for the diagnosis of acute appendicitis in everyday practice.

CEUS can play a role in helping the detection of the real extent of pericolic and distant abscesses: the purulent collection will not be enhanced, while inflamed tissues will be.

10.3.4 Ischemic Vs. Infectious Colitis

In daily practice, it is a relatively common dilemma to differentiate between ischemic colitis and infectious colitis. Even contrast-enhanced CT scan, which is considered the gold-standard imaging, can sometimes be unhelpful in providing a definitive diagnosis. B-mode US can detect a thickened colonic wall over a bowel segment longer than 10 cm, but findings are often not specific for accurate discrimination. In these cases, CEUS reveals itself as an easy and quick tool for ruling-out ischemic colitis.

Using a convex probe—the linear probe, though the right one for bowel exploration, is rarely set for CEUS—you scan the pathological segment of the large bowel (usually the descending colon). Be sure not to move the probe while waiting for the contrast enhancement. Ideally, it would be better to have a dual real-time visualization of both the B-mode and CEUS images on screen. Ask your co-worker to inject the contrast media (e.g., for SonoVue®, 2.4 mL bolus followed by 10 mL of saline solution) and wait.

After a few seconds (generally, 15–30 s), the large bowel wall should begin taking up the contrast, starting from the submucosal layer. If this is the case, then this is not an ischemic colitis! It could be infectious (Fig. 10.1).

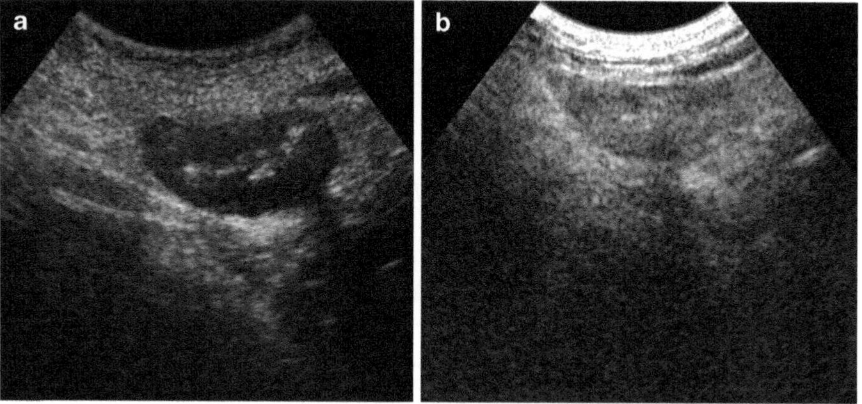

Fig. 10.1 Infectious colitis. (**a**) B-mode, transversal view of a thickened left colon, painful on graded compression. Findings could be compatible with both ischemic and infectious colitis. (**b**) after intravenous contrast media (SonoVue®), CEUS shows enhancement of the colonic wall. Ischemic colitis is ruled out

On the contrary, if the bowel wall remains hypoechoic: (1) be sure you did not move the probe from the right place; (2) slide the probe over a part of the colon you previously checked as normal (usually, the distal sigmoid loop) and verify if the segment wall there takes up contrast; (3) reassess the pathological segment in B-mode: stand still with the probe, turn on the machine contrast software and dual-image visualization, and inject the second half of the contrast solution (i.e., the remaining 2.4 mL bolus for SonoVue®). If still unenhanced, the colonic wall is ischemic. Now, the next right step is probably a contrast-enhanced CT in order to properly assess the extent of the ischemic colon and possible complications.

Remember!

- Contrast-specific software must be installed on the US equipment: Not every probe might be supported!
- CEUS software is generally available on convex probes. Do not worry about the possible related minor resolution: CEUS is based on "black-and-white" concept, findings are not limited using convex probes!

Appendix: Chapter 9—Test Yourself (Answers in the Appendix at the End of the Book)

Q1—CEUS is possible…

- On any US equipment with a convex probe.
- If you have the software on the US equipment.
- Only with the linear probe.

Further Reading

Atkinson NSS, Bryant RV, Dong Y, Maaser C, Kucharzik T, Maconi G, et al. How to perform gastrointestinal ultrasound: anatomy and normal findings. World J Gastroenterol. 2017;23(38):6931–41. https://doi.org/10.3748/wjg.v23.i38.6931.

Beckmann S, Simanowski JH. Update in contrast-enhanced ultrasound. Visc Med. 2020;36(6):476–86. https://doi.org/10.1159/000511352.

Cozzi D, Agostini S, Bertelli E, Galluzzo M, Papa E, Scevola G, et al. Contrast-Enhanced Ultrasound (CEUS) in Non-Traumatic Abdominal Emergencies. Ultrasound Int Open. 2020;6(3):E76–86. https://doi.org/10.1055/a-1347-5875.

Dirks K, et al. EFSUMB position paper: recommendations for gastrointestinal ultrasound (GIUS) in acute appendicitis and diverticulitis. Ultraschall Med. 2019;40:163–75.

Hamada T, Yamauchi M, Tanaka M, Hashimoto Y, Nakai K, Suenaga K. Prospective evaluation of contrast-enhanced ultrasonography with advanced dynamic flow for the diagnosis of intestinal ischaemia. Br J Radiol. 2007;80(956):603–8. https://doi.org/10.1259/bjr/59793102.

Hata J, Kamada T, Haruma K, Kusunoki H. Evaluation of bowel ischemia with contrast-enhanced US: initial experience. Radiology. 2005;236(2):712–5. https://doi.org/10.1148/radiol.2362040299.

Incesu L, Yazicioglu AK, Selcuk MB, Ozen N. Contrast-enhanced power Doppler US in the diagnosis of acute appendicitis. Eur J Radiol. 2004;50(2):201–9. https://doi.org/10.1016/S0720-048X(03)00102-5.

Medellin A, Merrill C, Wilson SR. Role of contrast-enhanced ultrasound in evaluation of the bowel. Abdom Radiol (NY). 2018;43(4):918–33. https://doi.org/10.1007/s00261-017-1399-6.

Mostbeck G, Adam EJ, Nielsen MB, Claudon M, Clevert D, Nicolau C, et al. How to diagnose acute appendicitis: ultrasound first. Insights Imaging. 2016;7(2):255–63. https://doi.org/10.1007/s13244-016-0469-6.

Quaia E, Migaleddu V, Baratella E, Pizzolato R, Rossi A, Grotto M, et al. The diagnostic value of small bowel wall vascularity after sulfur hexafluoride-filled microbubble injection in patients with Crohn's disease. Correlation with the therapeutic effectiveness of specific anti-inflammatory treatment. Eur J Radiol. 2009;69(3):438–44. https://doi.org/10.1016/j.ejrad.2008.10.029.

Chapter 11
FAST and E-FAST Protocols in Acute Abdomen: Something Heretical?

Luca Ponchietti, Carlos Yánez Benítez, Efterpi Chouridou, Diego Mariani, Alessia Malagnino, and Mauro Zago

Abbreviations

apm	Acts per minute
BE	Base Excess
bpm	Beats per minute
CRP	C-reactive protein
CT	Computed Tomography
E-FAST	Extended Focused Assessment with Sonography for Trauma
ER	Emergency room
FAST	Focused Assessment with Sonography for Trauma
Hb	Hemoglobin
HR	Heart rate
OR	Operating room

L. Ponchietti (✉) · C. Yánez Benítez
Department of General Surgery, San Jorge University Hospital, Huesca, Spain
e-mail: lponchietti@salud.aragon.es

E. Chouridou
General Surgeon for UNMISS (United Nations Mission in South Sudan), UN House Clinic, Juba, South Sudan

D. Mariani
ASST OVEST Milanese, General Surgery Department, ASST Ovest Milanese, "Ospedale Nuovo" di Legnano, Milano, Italy

A. Malagnino · M. Zago
General and Emergency Surgery Unit, General Surgery Department, A. Manzoni Hospital, Lecco, Italy

M. Zago et al. (eds.), *Point-of-care US for Acute Abdomen*,
https://doi.org/10.1007/978-3-031-40231-9_11

RR	Respiratory rate
SBP	Systolic blood pressure
SpO_2	Oxygen saturation
WBC	White Blood Cells

11.1 Introduction

The acute abdomen is a broad term describing a wide range of pathologies that present with a narrow spectrum of severe symptoms. The main surgical pathologies of the acute abdomen are appendicitis, cholecystitis, pancreatitis, diverticulitis, intestinal obstruction, and mesenteric vascular occlusion. The greatest number of patients, though, will be classified as non-specific abdominal pain, meaning that the clinical examination and the basic workflow (usually blood tests and simple X-rays) have not been able to orient toward a pathology, nor have warranted the request of an ultrasound (US) or a CT scan.

Considering that the exact etiology is not always immediately obvious and that the overall morbidity and mortality of acute abdomen are generally high, it is evident how the ability to quickly identify the subgroup of patients more at risk of complications or with a more evolved condition is paramount.

Probably, the only good thing which almost all abdominal emergencies have in common is that independent of the cause, as the case gets more "severe," there is an accumulation of fluid. This fluid can be reactive or exudative, can be sterile or infected or even blood, depending on the pathology. Whatever its characteristics, when it reaches a sufficient amount, it can be seen by US. For these reasons, it seems logical to use the same technique used in trauma patients, E-FAST, in acute non-traumatic abdominal pain to rule-out or rule-in the presence of free fluid (FF). Furthermore, the possibility to assess the pleural cavity for free fluid or pneumothorax can add useful information in the acute abdominal pain.

It is not the purpose of this book to go through the technique and clinical findings of an E-FAST study, that have been already discussed elsewhere. Instead, we will propose a clinical-oriented discussion on how a positive or a negative E-FAST may change your approach in any patient with acute abdominal pain.

First of all, it is essential to consider how much FF can be detected by abdominal US. Everyday practice and clinical studies provide various estimates being the minimum amount of FF detectable from as low as 10 cc to as high as 600 cc. Many of these studies were done on trauma patients, and many of them used old-technologies machines and probes. Erring on the safe side, we may safely say that we can have a positive FAST with a minimum of 300 mL of FF when using a curvilinear, low-frequency (usually 1–8 MHz) probe. These concepts appear essential for our discussion. You don't use linear, high-frequency probes—they may detect even small amounts of FF that, in some cases, can be considered physiologic/normal (e.g., ovulating female). As in trauma patients, we look for gross amounts of blood (not single blood cells!), when performing an E-FAST in the patient with acute abdominal pain we look for gross amounts of FF. Remember that the aim of the exam is just the assessment of the presence or absence of intra-abdominal or intra-thoracic FF, not a complete anatomical examination of the contents of these cavities. For comparative purposes, imagine making a quick US assessment of a tank filled with water: E-FAST will only tell you only if the tank is full or empty. It does not assess whether on the inside there is a cute goldfish or a piranha swimming in the water or, if it is empty, if there is a snail or a scorpion on the ground.

In case of a patient with acute abdomen, the presence or absence of FF on E-FAST will give you only one more information, to be integrated into the whole clinical picture as to help out your decision-making process. One of the subtle differences between non-emergency doctors and emergency doctors (and particularly surgeons) is the appreciation of the value of both "ruling-out" and "ruling-in" a condition. Clinicians, and all the non-emergency community, have been trained to reach a diagnosis. This usually starts with several differential diagnoses, and progressively narrows until reaching the good one. These "narrowing down" can be achieved in many ways, and in most cases is time consuming. It indeed seems to provide great joy to them, which is reflected in lengthy clinical entries.

This philosophy clashes with that of emergency doctors/surgeons who, without any exception, worry basically about knowing if the patient needs an operation straight away (in the first 6 h), without time for a preoperative optimization, or if their condition allows for a less aggressive management. Any non-traumatic condition that needs to be operated during the first 6 h is usually bad for the patient, and it commonly carries higher mortality and morbidity. But these cases are also the ones who benefit the most from a prompt assessment of their severity and aggressive management.

These are the reasons why emergency doctors and surgeons, when called upon assessing an acute abdomen, as a rule are not only worried about knowing what the cause of the acute abdomen is. In fact, the main focus is to recognize how severely the physiological status has been affected and how quickly the workup needs to be done. Their fear is to underestimate a case and linger too much. At the same time, they are well aware that if the condition allows for preoperative optimization, it has to be done for the patient's sake.

According to Schein's *Common-Sense Emergency Abdominal Surgery*, acute abdomen can present as one of the following five clinical patterns:

- Abdominal pain and shock.
- Generalized peritonitis.
- Localized peritonitis.
- Intestinal obstruction.
- "Medical" illness.

We will show you briefly how E-FAST can find its place in the management of each of these patterns. We will initially consider the use of E-FAST in modern healthcare systems, where formal radiology and CT scans are readily available. Lastly, we will describe the benefits of E-FAST in low-resources healthcare systems (*that may also be your own hospital during the night, if the radiologist is not on shift*), where US is going to likely be the only "radiological" equipment available.

11.1.1 Sudden Abdominal Pain and Shock

Depending on the patient's age and sex, the pattern "sudden abdominal pain and shock" usually rhymes with ruptured abdominal aortic aneurysm (AAA) or ectopic pregnancy. These patients need to be quickly assessed, and surgical treatment is the only available option when comorbidities and severity allow it. An E-FAST (a non-anatomic examination of the abdomen) is quite useful to help you make the correct decision in such dramatic scenarios.

For example, in the young female patient, FF presence will promptly confirm the diagnosis. This is a rule-in situation because we find the expected finding. Conversely, in the same situation, a negative E-FAST is not able per se to help you reach a diagnosis. However, it will most likely convince you to start aggressive non-surgical management while requesting more tests because you have ruled-out hemoperitoneum.

In the older population presenting with shock preceded by sudden abdominal pain, E-FAST alone is, unfortunately, of a more limited utility. A positive E-FAST does not help in ruling out other non-surgical causes of this clinical pattern, nor a negative E-FAST helps you ruling out a retroperitoneal hematoma. To be pragmatic, to assess this second group of patients with US, you need to learn some more skills, fundamentally how to assess the aorta. If the aorta is normal, ruptured AAA can be excluded. E-FAST alone can lead you nowhere.

Another clinical syndrome that can present with acute sudden abdominal pain and shock is visceral perforation, particularly peptic ulcer perforation. Even in this case, the immediate detection of abdominal FF on E-FAST gives you a quick confirmation of your suspicions, far before the results of lab tests, standard (and often not useful) abdominal plain film, and eventually a CT scan. Moreover, adding a simple US-guided maneuver, you could retrieve a sample of the fluid through an US-guided Diagnostic Peritoneal Aspiration (DPA): if it is green or brown, you can readily make your diagnosis and finalize your decisions. You could probably skip any other imaging and proceed to emergency surgery.

To summarize, the role of the E-FAST in a fertile woman in shock after a sudden onset of acute abdominal pain is to confirm the (quite obvious) diagnosis. It takes almost no time to be performed. In case of a negative E-FAST, which is utterly an uncommon situation, it brings a sort of relief, giving time for a more detailed workup. All in all, it is highly recommended to E-FAST these patients.

In the older population, E-FAST alone is of limited use because it is not able to rule-in or rule-out ruptured AAA, nor the need for emergency surgery (rushing to theatre), nor the feasibility of a less aggressive management. If you are not trained in assessing the aorta, think twice about using your E-FAST findings to guide the management of these patients. In the suspicion of visceral perforation, FAST views allow you to search the first finding of hollow viscus perforation, which is FF. Putting your US findings together with the patient's medical history and possibly the results of a DPA, you will probably have enough for speeding up your decision-making process.

11.1.2 Generalized Peritonitis and Localized Peritonitis

For the purposes of this chapter, these two clinical patterns will be discussed together. We have been taught that the diagnosis and the distinction between the two are clinical. First, the patient has a history of worsening abdominal pain and shows signs of sepsis (note the difference with "sudden" abdominal pain and shock). If the abdominal pain is confined to one quadrant of the abdomen, and at exploration you can elicit signs of peritonitis (namely, defense and rebound tenderness) confined to one quadrant, you diagnose a localized peritonitis. When the pain and same clinical signs are found in all the quadrants of the abdomen, you diagnose a generalized peritonitis. No need to say that localized peritonitis usually shows fewer symptoms and mild signs of sepsis, while generalized peritonitis is almost invariantly a much more severe situation.

Sometimes, however, clinical signs can underestimate the severity of the peritonitis: what seems to be a localized peritonitis, it is not actually. It is not uncommon to find diffuse peritonitis in patients clinically diagnosed with localized peritonitis, such for example those with acute appendicitis or acute diverticulitis.

On the contrary, it is unfortunately relatively common to find diffuse peritonitis in patients with mild or no clinical signs at all. Indeed, the frequent use (and abuse) of painkillers, as well some medical conditions (e.g., diabetes, dementia), can alter the perception of pain. In addition, sometimes the clinical picture is far worse than the actual findings, as for example in case of acute pancreatitis.

Now, all things considered, let's see some practical examples and evaluate what the US probe can add to the clinical and physical examination.

It is 11.00 p.m., and you are assessing a young man with acute abdominal pain whose characteristics are highly suggestive of non-complicated acute appendicitis. Clinical examination shows mild systemic signs and localized peritonitis in the right lower quadrant. Blood tests are congruent with your diagnosis, meaning that you are not extremely worried by them. Alvarado score is 9 (i.e., high probability of acute appendicitis), Appendicitis Inflammatory Response (AIR) score is 8 (i.e., indeterminate risk).

This seems an all-too-common emergency. In most institutions, you will wait until the next morning to decide whether to go directly to the OR or request an US/CT scan to confirm your diagnosis. This is what you do in real life in a modern health system.

Now, imagine doing an US scan at 11 p.m.: if you have read Chap. 6 on acute appendicitis, you know how to detect a pathological appendix. Congratulations! Moreover, if no FF is shown on abdominal E-FAST views (*rule-out*), you can be confident in your diagnosis since you have not found signs of diffuse peritonitis or pelvic collections.

On the other hand, if you found FF in the pouch of Douglas or the Morrison, probably you will change your attitude (*rule-in*) as this would no longer be a probable non-complicated acute appendicitis. If you're not confident enough or if you can't find the appendix, you will probably need to request a formal US or a CT scan, and maybe you will have to go to OR overnight because your patient is not as well as he seemed to be.

Imagine another patient, let's say a 60-year-old woman with acute abdomen and type-II diabetes. The pain started in the left lower quadrant, the exploration shows mild diffuse pain, with no rebound tenderness. Her vitals are normal. Blood tests are almost unremarkable: mild chronic renal failure, just a little bit of WBC elevation, CRP minimally raised.

Let's be honest: all in all, she is not that sick, and you are really not that worried. It is 2 a.m., and you think of giving her painkillers, I.V. fluids, and re-evaluate in the morning. This appears like the most correct thing to do.

But imagine again you use your US probe to perform an E-FAST. If your examination is negative (i.e., no FF), you are comforted in your decision. Whatever is her problem, the absence of FF rules out bowel suffering or diffuse peritonitis. But if you see a tiny band of FF in the pelvis and Morrison, well… We are sure that you will get your patient a CT scan straight away, and this may lead to a diagnosis of Hinchey 3 acute diverticulitis (although, if you have read the dedicated Chap. 5, you may be able to reach this diagnosis by US without the need for a CT scan…).

We are sure these two clinical cases bring back many memories to all of us. We are also optimistic that you have started appreciating the utility of E-FAST in non-trauma patients.

This is why we strongly recommend to "at least" perform an E-FAST in all patients with acute abdominal pain. In a few minutes, you can easily rule out or rule in signs of acute peritonitis, independently of its origin, and this will determine a better management of your cases.

11.1.3 Intestinal Obstruction

You all know that there are many causes of intestinal obstruction and how to do the workup. With a FAST you can only detect FF as an indirect sign of bowel suffering. It is quick and easy to do and it can help you request a CT scan sooner than later. Even if you will not indicate a surgical approach based on a positive FAST alone, the crucial information it easily provides makes it always worthy to perform it. If you feel confident, an US-guided DPA could help you to rule-in bowel suffering: if the aspirated fluid is serosanguineous, you probably must speed up your decision-making process.

11.1.4 "Medical" Illness

Most common causes of false abdominal pain are myocardial infarction, basal pneumonia, ketoacidosis, plus many other conditions that you will never see during your years as doctors.

Even though a pleural effusion could be considered maybe as an indirect sign of basal pneumonia, we don't want to fool you. E-FAST has realistically little use in these cases.

11.1.5 Monitoring of Postoperative Course and Complications

US and E-FAST views can play a pivotal role in speeding up the assessment and management of operated patients with a not ordinary postoperative course. Whenever you have a doubt of possible intra-abdominal complications, you would like to have the possibility of taking a "look" inside, wouldn't you? In most cases, you will rely on lab test results, and you may ask for a CT scan. However, if you know how to use a US probe, why don't put it on the belly and have that "look" inside?

Let's imagine some possible real-life case scenarios.

You're on the night shift. The day before, your colleagues performed an elective laparoscopic cholecystectomy in a 35-year-old female. Surgical procedure was reported uneventful, lasting about 30 min skin-to-skin. Now, the ward nurse calls you because the patient is sweating and a little bit agitated. Her vitals are as follows: SBP 110 mmHg, HR 80 bpm, RR 18 apm, SpO_2 95% in room air. Physical abdominal examination is not significant. What to think? Biliary fistula? Bleeding? … Anxious patient?

You ask for urgent blood tests and meanwhile you increase fluid infusion rate, asking the nurse to call you once lab tests are ready. After half an hour, here are the results: Hb 12 g/L (preoperative value: 13 g/L), WBC 13,500/mcL, Lactates 2 mmol/L, BE −2 mEq/L. All in all, these results are inconclusive; moreover, the patient is now feeling better, not sweating. You decide to monitor the patient and repeat blood samples at 4–6 h.

However, 2 h later you are paged in again as the patient is once more feeling unwell and sweating. She is hypotensive (SBP 95 mmHg) and tachycardic (HR 105 bpm). Remembering our previous recommendation, you decide to perform a bedside FAST. The image you see is reported in Fig. 11.1: a large amount of FF consistent with hemoperitoneum. For sure, you now know what to do, but maybe a FAST scan performed 2 h before may have changed early on your decision-making process, don't you think?

Here is another case. A 76-year-old man on third postoperative day after right hepatectomy is dyspneic and slightly febrile (37.4 °C). Labs: WBC 11,800/mcL, CRP 12 mg/L, liver enzymes within normal range.

Aware of the previous experience, you decide to immediately perform a bedside E-FAST. What do you see? Look at Fig. 11.2: now it is up to you to decide whether to drain or not the pleural effusion right away. In any case, you now know the reason for his dyspnea.

We are sure you face plenty of similar situations in your everyday practice: ruling-in or ruling-out FF with a quick US assessment can often give you the background you need to speed up treatment, call for help, decide for a "wait-and-see"

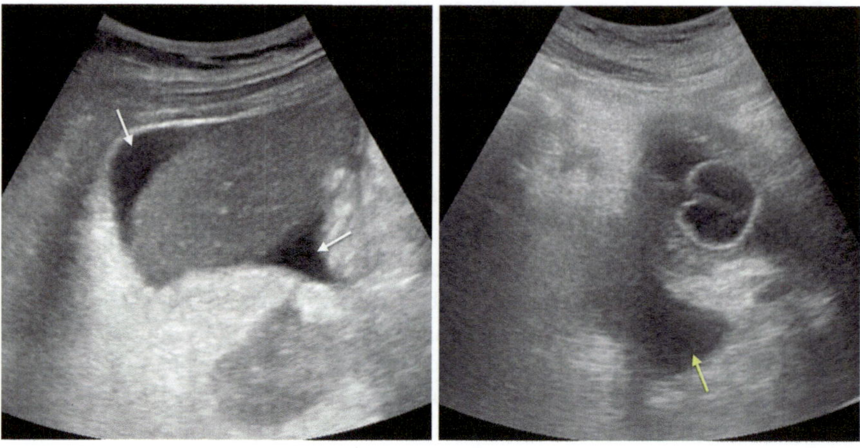

Fig. 11.1 Large amount of free fluid in the right upper quadrant (perihepatic and Morrison pouch, *white arrows*) and pelvis (behind the Foley balloon, *yellow arrow*). Do you agree that the patient is bleeding?

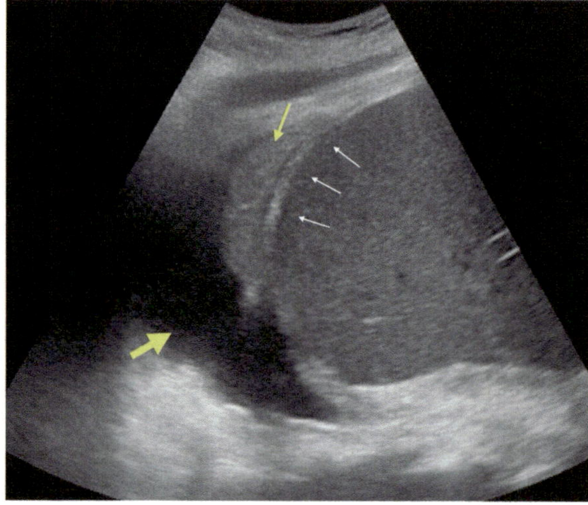

Fig. 11.2 Significant right pleural effusion (*bold yellow arrows*), with atelectasis of the right lower lobe (*thin yellow arrow*), cranially to the diaphragm (*white arrows*). To drain or not to drain?

approach, etc. This is not always true, of course: if US examination is negative, constantly ask yourself whether this finding is enough, or if you need to repeat it or to go on with further imaging.

11.1.6 Limited Resources

Let's not fool ourselves. Apart from unstable trauma patients, we are CT-dependent for many of our medical decisions. Also, it is not so uncommon to be called to assess a patient after an extensive workup has already been done (including, of course, the CT scan). We can have lengthy discussions on whether this is good practice or not and whether this is cost-effective or not. Undoubtedly, the liberal use of CT scan makes our lives easier, and it is often safer for the patients. Also, there is no turning back.

Unfortunately, most of the world population cannot benefit from the resources that in richer countries are commonly available. In many places, surgeons and clinicians still assess their patients and decide with the clinical findings alone or with little more than simple blood tests and simple radiographies. Moreover, patients in these settings arrive quite late to the ER (lack of transportation or of trust in "official" medicine), after having consumed a great quantity of painkillers, which consequently leads to the absence of clinical symptoms, especially when the presence of other diseases (such as diabetes), that may alter the clinical image, are unknown to the patient. Language barriers and cultural differences may also produce a very confusing result, where the patient's history is unknown, clinical signs are controversial or conflicting, and communication between physician and patient is difficult, if not impossible. For all these reasons, an "objective tool" is needed, when facing the possibility of an acute abdomen, in order to clarify whether the patient is in need of an operation soon or a conservative treatment would be more appropriate.

In these scenarios, it is clear how being able to detect FF in a patient with an acute abdomen is useful in guiding your clinical decisions. Regarding gynecological emergencies, ectopic pregnancy is quite frequent in these settings, due to limited use or presence of Ante-Natal Programs. In these cases, FAST is being performed almost simultaneously with the clinical examination, even before receiving blood for tests, and the patient can be led to the OR immediately. Regarding the suspicion of generalized peritonitis, blood tests to verify sepsis are usually not available, and if the clinical examination is confusing, as mentioned before, the presence of FF in the abdomen can make the difference in the treatment of the patient. Repeated ultrasounds may be needed, as situation evolves, and an extra knowledge of scanning the abdomen can be helpful to make a diagnosis prior to the operation (e.g., appendicitis, cholecystitis, diverticulitis), even though the sole presence of FF can be conclusive for the need of an operation. Finally, if an intestinal obstruction is suspected, the presence of FF detected by FAST, should alert you of the possibility of bowel suffering and make you consider surgical management. In these cases, the patient is usually entering a high dependency unit and is more closely observed until a final decision for an operation is taken. But, in precarious situations, surgical approach can be sometimes more aggressive and earlier, due to lack of other tests, and therefore FF detection by FAST views and its increase in quantity can sometimes be the only indication for operation.

Using US in limited resources settings encounters its challenges. Most probably, the only US machine available will be a small, portable one, with old software and no possibility of printing. The images that can be received will not be as sophisticated as those from a modern US machine. Therefore, in these situations, it is highly advisable to start using your machine as often as possible, even when you are certain there is no FF in the abdomen or other pathology/condition to detect. Patients always appreciate a thorough doctor, anyway. This constant practice with your equipment will teach you how to recognize the normal images, using old hardware and software, and will help you when you will get the real pathological images.

On the other hand, patients in these settings tend to arrive generally late to the ER. Therefore, an "ultrasound-inexperienced" emergency physician or surgeon will easily identify the bigger amount of FF already collected in the abdomen.

Once more, let us also remember that, even in high- or middle-income countries, the presence of radiologists is not assured 24/7 in many hospitals: getting basics but essential US findings can change the path and the outcome of your patients.

11.2 Conclusions

The early detection of intra-abdominal fluid by the abdominal E-FAST views in patients with non-traumatic abdominal pain must be an alert sign in relation to the severity of the acute abdomen. This finding can contribute to confirming clinical suspicion and help the surgeon in the process of guiding pre-surgical workup and, depending on the clinical situation of the patient, even decide immediate surgical management.

Although not a replacement for the more sensitive imaging studies or focused clinical US, as a rapid, non-invasive test it has significant advantages that have been extensively proven through its use in trauma. The average time to perform an E-FAST by an experienced operator is 2–3 min. At the same time, it must be remembered that E-FAST is a screening test, and false-negative and false-positive examinations can occur.

FAST is easy to perform because it does not look at the abdominal structures, only at the presence or absence of FF. Its success in trauma is because in an unstable trauma patient it gives you all the information you need to know to decide whether or not the patient needs to be brought straight to the OR. In non-trauma patients, unfortunately, it has many shortcomings. To rule-out or rule-in FF is useful, but realistically, if you plan to do an US to your patients with an acute abdomen, we are sure that you will want to first learn some basics of abdominal US to answer your clinical queries. It is not difficult to learn how to scan an aorta, a gallbladder, an appendix, or a kidney. Once you have gained these skills, yes, you will have a very powerful tool in your hands.

In addition, what appeals the most is the possibility to introduce E-FAST as a triage tool for nurses or paramedics. Used by non-doctors, a patient with abdominal pain and FF should prompt a quicker hospital referral or medical examination because they are potentially suffering from a more severe condition.

Tips and Tricks

- Scan systematically and thoroughly
- Use the urine in the bladder to set your machine: free fluid has usually the same echogenicity… but remember: serosanguineous and enteric fluids could appear hyperechogenic as well!
- E-FAST is a dynamic evaluation: repeat it at different moments, whenever you need!

Red Flags

- *Pitfall*: linear high-frequency probes can easily detect small amounts of fluids that may be physiological/normal. Be aware of the clinics!
- *Warning*: pay attention when E-FAST is performed in patients with peritoneal dialysis, cirrhosis, known ascites, carcinomatosis

Remember!

- The presence of free intra-abdominal fluid could mean bowel suffering, peritonitis, or bowel perforation: rule out each and every one of these hypotheses!
- The absence of free fluid does not rule out a severe abdominal condition. On the other hand, the presence of free fluid needs to be contextualized with the current clinical picture
- *Be liberal with DPA*: when in doubt, retrieve a sample of fluid!

Appendix: Chapter 10—Test Yourself (Answers in the Appendix at the End of the Book)

Q1—Do you think E-FAST views can be useful for a right decision-making process in a wide range of situations outside of trauma settings?

- Yes.
- No.

Further Reading

Abrams BJ, Sukumvanich P, Seibel R, Moscati R, Jehle D. Ultrasound for the detection of intraperitoneal fluid: the role of Trendelenburg positioning. Am J Emerg Med. 1999;17(2):117–20. https://doi.org/10.1016/s0735-6757(99)90040-2.

AIUM practice parameter for the performance of the focused assessment with sonography for trauma (FAST) examination - American Institute of Ultrasound in Medicine; 2014.

Alex Ng - The FAST examination. How good is FAST? Trauma.org. 2001;6:12. http://www.trauma.org/radiology/FASThowgood.htm.

Branney SW, Wolfe RE, Moore EE, Albert NP, Heinig M, Mestek M, et al. Quantitative sensitivity of ultrasound in detecting free intraperitoneal fluid. J Trauma. 1995;39(2):375–80. https://doi.org/10.1097/00005373-199508000-00032.

Cartwright SL, Knudson MP. Diagnostic imaging of acute abdominal pain in adults. Am Fam Physician. 2015;91(7):452–9.

Commissioning guide: Emergency general surgery (acute abdominal pain) - Association of Surgeons of Great Britain and Ireland (ASGBI); 2014.

Dietrich CF, Mathis G, Blaivas M, Volpicelli G, Seibel A, Wastl D, et al. Lung B-line artefacts and their use. J Thorac Dis. 2016;8(6):1356–65. https://doi.org/10.21037/jtd.2016.04.55.

Forsby J, Henriksson L. Detectability of intraperitoneal fluid by ultrasonography. An experimental investigation. Acta Radiol Diagn (Stockh). 1984;25(5):375–8. https://doi.org/10.1177/028418518402500505.

Raman S, Somasekar K, Winter RK, Lewis MH. Are we overusing ultrasound in non-traumatic acute abdominal pain? Postgrad Med J. 2004;80(941):177–9. https://doi.org/10.1136/pgmj.2003.013805.

Schein M, Rogers PN. Schein's common sense emergency abdominal surgery. Berlin: Springer-Verlag; 2005. https://doi.org/10.1007/b138098.

Chapter 12
Cost-Effectiveness of Clinical Ultrasound in Acute Abdomen

Alessia Malagnino, Giorgia Pezzotta, Samantha Bozzo, Giuliano Masiero, Diego Mariani, and Mauro Zago

12.1 Introduction

Patients presenting with urgent symptoms usually require immediate diagnosis and treatment. Due to its portability, lower costs, and lack of exposure to ionizing radiation, ultrasound (US) imaging has been increasingly applied for evaluation of acute clinical problems. The consequent widespread use of clinical US among non-radiologists has determined a new perspective in the timing of treatment and management of patients, particularly in acute care settings. For these reasons, the practice of clinical US should be analyzed also from an economic point of view, especially when considering public health resources.

In this chapter, we aimed to answer the following questions:

- Are there economic benefits from performing US as a first clinical assessment for acute abdomen, in addition to the already described medical issues?

A. Malagnino (✉) · S. Bozzo · M. Zago
General and Emergency Surgery Unit, General Surgery Department, ASST Lecco, "A. Manzoni" Hospital, Lecco, Italy
e-mail: ag.malagnino@asst-lecco.it

G. Pezzotta
Department of Management, Information and Production Engineering, University of Bergamo, Bergamo, Italy

G. Masiero
Department of Economics (DSE), University of Bergamo, Bergamo, Italy

D. Mariani
ASST OVEST Milanese, General Surgery Department, Ospedale di Legnano, Milano, Italy

M. Zago et al. (eds.), *Point-of-care US for Acute Abdomen*,
https://doi.org/10.1007/978-3-031-40231-9_12

- Can point-of-care US (POCUS) make possible to reduce costs derived from days of hospitalization, expensive and radiation-emitting procedures, and maybe even inappropriate hospital admissions and/or surgical interventions?

12.2 Literature Data

The cost-benefit of using US for diagnosis and evaluation of abnormal conditions has already been established in a variety of situations. An American study demonstrated that in patients with musculoskeletal disorders the use of US rather than MR imaging determined a saving of nearly 7 billion dollars. An Italian study on the use of lung US in the intensive care unit demonstrated that an average higher number of chest X-rays was performed when US was not applied (i.e., 0.97 vs. 0.42 exams per patients), and the reported estimated cost-reduction rate after introduction of lung US was 57%.

The cost-effectiveness analyses have also considered the equality and/or superiority of US compared to other imaging methods in terms of accuracy and efficiency. For example, a recent meta-analysis determined that bedside US yielded a mean sensitivity of 90% and a mean specificity of 95% in detecting acute appendicitis.

Likewise, US presents greater accuracy in revealing lung contusion than standard chest X-ray, and it is as accurate as CT scan with the advantages that it is easier to perform, it is radiation-free, and does not require the patient to be moved. US is also an effective tool in the diagnosis of pneumothorax, and it has been shown to be as accurate as lung CT scan at providing additional information pertaining to the extension of disease compared with chest X-rays. In addition, a recent paper analyzing the impact of bedside US, performed by trained physicians in an elderly population of an Internal Medicine ward, showed POCUS reduces standard radiological and US examinations in these settings.

Nevertheless, there is currently poor data on cost-effectiveness and economic impact of clinical US in acute abdomen. We believe its role should be emphasized, particularly with reference to administration of health resources. Considering the topics displayed in the previous chapters, it appears quite clear how the US evaluation of the patient can be a helpful tool in the decision-making process. Focused and "on-the-go" images of the affected organs, as well as the possibility of getting biological samples through interventional ultrasound-guided maneuvers, represent a significant addition to the patient's history, signs, and symptoms, allowing the doctor to outline earlier—and often more easily—a diagnosis, and decide for hospital admission, further investigation, need for surgery, or even discharge.

12.2.1 Some Additional Data

The interest of the authors for the cost-benefit and economic impact of surgeon-performed POCUS (SP-POCUS) is long-lasting. In a prospective series of 100 patients, we were able to demonstrate that, after a short specific training and following a precise protocol, E-FAST allowed to safely skip chest X-rays during primary survey of trauma patients, thus reducing time for evaluation and treatment. This did not only have a clinical effect, reducing morbidity and mortality, but from an economical point of view entailed a significant saving of resources (mainly, working time).

In another retrospective analysis, we compared the rate of negative appendectomies (i.e., not confirmed on histologic examination) in a single referral center over a period of 1 year. In this case series, we analyzed the results of two groups of surgeons, one performing SP-POCUS and the other one not. Overall, the rates of requested CT-scan and negative appendectomies were significantly lower for those surgeons performing SP-POCUS (Table 12.1). The mean difference in the diagnostic cost per patient between the two groups was 257.82 € ($p < 0.01$).

12.3 An Original Study

It would be of interest to briefly report our experience at a single, non-trauma, General Surgery department in the Milan metropolitan area, where we carried out a prospective evaluation of the impact of SP-POCUS on decision-making processes, as well as its implications in terms of organizational and economic issues.

Between 2015 and 2019, a prospective registry was established to register all the POCUS performed at our Institution, including clinical data, derived diagnosis, decision-making processes, and organizational effects. During the study period, 1232 SP-POCUS were recorded, and the procedures were performed by a surgical team where only 3 surgeons out of 9 were trained in POCUS examination. Overall, 95% of POCUS were performed for non-trauma reasons. In 13.3% of cases, bedside US was indicated to assess and manage postoperative course and complications; in 7% of cases, US was used to manage pneumothorax and pleural effusions; in 21.8% of cases, US was useful for diagnostic/therapeutic interventional procedures.

Table 12.1 Rates of CT scan and negative appendectomies between patients treated by surgeons trained at performing SP-POCUS and those treated by surgeons not trained at performing SP-POCUS

	CT scan (%)	Negative appendectomy (%)
US-trained surgeons	18/202 (*8.9%*)	3/202 (*1.5%*)
Not US-trained surgeons	24/39 (*61.5%*)	4/39 (*10.2%*)
	$p < 0.001$	**$p < 0.003$**

SP-POCUS allowed to shorten time-to-clinical-decision (TCD) in 20.8% of cases, and it impacted in saving-of-further-imaging (SFI) in 16% of cases.

A preliminary cost-benefit analysis was conducted over a sample of the entire registry, namely SP-POCUS performed between 2018 and 2019. We carried out a clinical trial on the assessment of patients with acute signs and symptoms of thoracic and/or abdominal disorders, and we analyzed the performance of the surgical team, encompassing both ultrasound-skilled and non-ultrasound-skilled surgeons. For the initial assessment, patients were submitted to either bedside surgeon-performed US or other radiological examination (i.e., radiologist-performed US, chest X-ray, CT scan, MR imaging), depending on the surgeon on duty, as well as on the clinical onset and patient characteristics. Overall, US was the most performed exam both in adults and in youngest patients.

The mean estimated time for performance of clinical US by surgeons was about 8 min, which considers the time required for machinery transport and setting, the time for actual US assessment, and the time for reporting the examination. Conversely, the mean estimated time for the performance of a chest X-ray, a radiologist-performed US, or a contrast-enhanced CT scan was 31, 33, and 62 min, respectively. These intervals consider the time for preparing, moving, and transporting the patient back and forth to the radiology department, as well as the time for carrying out and reporting the examination, plus a latency period before the report reading by the surgeon. Of course, in these cases the intervals involve not only the surgeon, but also the radiologists, nurses, X-ray technicians, and other paramedical staff.

Over the 2-year study period, a total of 506 clinical US has been set up by surgeons on acute care patients, both in the emergency department and in the surgical ward. For the purposes of the study, the patients who had been "led on the way of radiology" at first glance (i.e., 19%) underwent a second-step clinical US as part of a single-blind control study.

Major clinical signs and/or suspicions prompting evaluation of acute care conditions by the surgical team are summarized in Fig. 12.1.

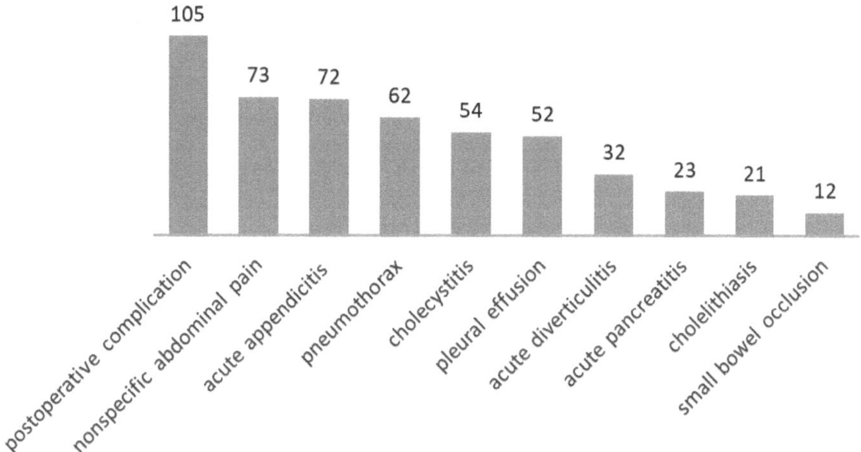

Fig. 12.1 Surgeon-performed clinical US according to clinical signs and/or suspicion

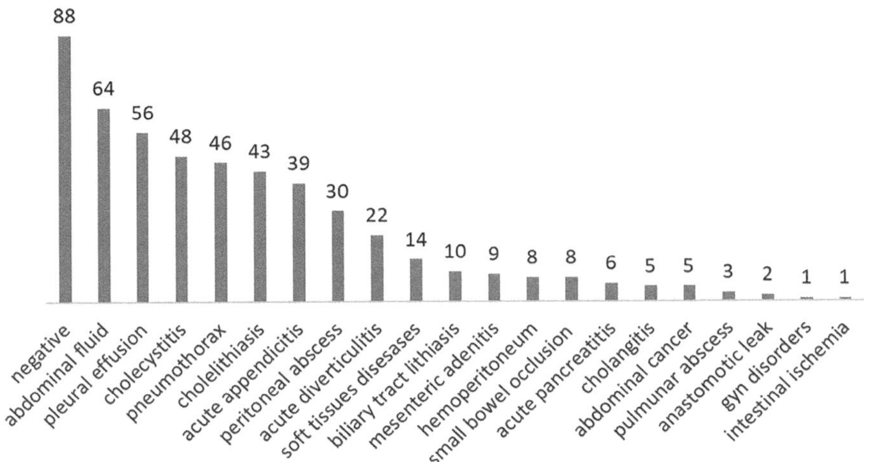

Fig. 12.2 Surgeon-performed clinical US according to US findings

Table 12.2 Decision-making after surgeon-performed clinical US

	n.	%
Conservative treatment	191	37.8
Discharge	48	9.5
Chest tube insertion	85	16.8
Chest tube removal	21	4.1
DPA (diagnostic peritoneal aspiration)	37	7.3
Emergency surgery	85	16.8
Elective surgery	11	2.2
Biopsy	7	1.4
Other examinations	21	4.1

The performance of clinical US allowed to make a diagnosis as well as to discriminate those requiring urgent/emergency treatment from those who needed further evaluations and/or less pressing inpatient treatments, as displayed in Fig. 12.2.

We then evaluated how performing a clinical US affected the decision-making process on patient's admission and management. Therefore, we determined what happened when clinical US was performed as a first step, and we tried to realistically figure out what could have happened if clinical US had always been performed as part of the initial assessment. Clinical and management outcomes resulting from receiving bedside US are shown in Table 12.2.

It should be underlined that 9.5% of cases were discharged after surgeon-performed US assessment, thus avoiding further useless examinations, inpatient treatments, and even surgery. Among those discharged after clinical US, 10 (20.8%) patients did not require admission to the surgical department and 12 (25.0%)

patients could have avoided being admitted if US had been carried out as part of the initial evaluation.

When considering the Diagnostic Related Group (DRG) refunds charged to the Italian National Health System (NHS) for those patients (mainly evaluated for acute appendicitis, acute diverticulitis, and acute cholecystitis), performing a clinical US resulted in a saving of about 19,300 € and further 24,100 € could have been potentially saved if US was carried out, for a total amount of 43,400 €.

For example, when analyzing patients with suspected acute appendicitis, which is one of the most frequent causes requiring surgical assessment, we recorded 72 suspected cases. Of these, only 39 (54%) patients were confirmed by clinical US. The current DRG refund charged to the Italian NHS for those operated on non-complicated acute appendicitis amounts to 2550 € for the whole hospital stay, to which an extra 200 € toll is charged per every day exceeding the trim point (i.e., 8 days). In the present analysis, clinical US would have avoided admission (either actual or potential) in 9 patients, determining a saving of about 23,000 €. It is also worth noting that all patients undergoing appendectomy after surgeon-performed US had the diagnosis confirmed on the surgical specimen.

We then assessed each case in terms of actual and potentially saved: days of hospital stay, number of radiological examinations performed (i.e., radiologist-performed US, chest X-ray, CT scan, MR imaging), surgical procedures performed, and other variables, such as indication to endoscopic procedures. Results are summarized in Tables 12.2 and 12.3.

Some other results and insights have been derived from this research, as outlined in the following paragraphs.

12.3.1 Days of Hospitalization

In Italy, the mean and median length of stay (LOS) for acute care patients are 6 and 4 days, respectively. Therefore, assuming a mean 6-day stay for the whole study population, it is possible to state that over the 2-year study period we managed to save 3% of total days of hospitalization and a further 2% could have been saved if clinical US had been performed as a first step at the time of initial assessment.

Table 12.3 Cost-effectiveness of clinical US for acute abdomen

	Actual savings (n)	*Potential savings (n)*
Days of hospitalization	94	59
Radiologist-performed US	24	10
Chest X-ray	75	10
CT scan	61	34
MR imaging	2	1
Operating room hours	22 (18 surgical procedures)	3 (3 surgical procedures)
Endoscopic examinations	5	0

Indeed, LOS is an important indicator of efficiency of hospital management. Reduction in LOS results in decreased risk of infection and medication side-effects, improvement in the quality of treatment, and increased hospital profit with more efficient bed management. Additionally, reduction in LOS has also a favorable impact on social and working issues related to hospitalization for both patients and their families.

12.3.2 Operating Room Hours

In the present analysis, a total of 245 (48.8%) patients underwent surgery before or after clinical US evaluation. Given the fact that by performing a clinical US assessment we have been able to avoid 18 surgical procedures, we can state that we saved the costs related to 7% of total surgery and a further 1.2% could have been saved if clinical US had been performed as a first step at the time of initial assessment. It goes without saying that the physical and psychological impact of surgery is remarkable, especially when avoidable.

12.3.3 Other Radiological and Endoscopic Investigations

As shown in Table 12.3, clinical US succeeded at avoiding (and could potentially have avoided) a significant amount of radiological and endoscopic investigations. This results in multiple cost-savings including: expenditure related to the performance of the examination, outflow of machinery and human resources, time spent for the whole procedure and for the transport of the patient, in addition to the possible discomfort related to the examination *per se*.

To give an idea of the amount of money potentially saved, we should consider that the mean Italian NHS fees provided for outpatient services are as follows: 60 € for an abdominal US, 15 € for a chest X-ray, 150 € for a contrast-enhanced CT scan of the abdomen, and 180 € for a contrast-enhanced MR imaging of the abdomen. For endoscopy, the current mean fees are 50 € for esophagogastroduodenoscopy and 80 € for colonoscopy. In addition, estimating the average time required for the whole performance of the radiological examinations in our sample population, we have been able to save about 116 h of personnel working time, compared to the 73 h required for clinical US ($\Delta = 43$ working hours).

12.4 Conclusions

Clinical US provides the ability to rapidly evaluate and diagnose a wide range of clinical abnormalities in almost every field of medicine. Compared to other imaging methods, clinical US determines an increased cost-efficiency and cost-benefit in the diagnosis and management of patients with thoracic and abdominal problems. It is portable, easy-to-perform, and radiation-free, and it results in significant lower costs in terms of both equipment and professionals involved. Further research and evaluations are required to provide appropriate optimization of patient care through analysis of costs, efficiency, experience, accuracy, disease states, and clinical outcomes. Focused training could be the key for getting a significant saving of healthcare resources as well.

Remember!
- *POCUS is cost-effective*
- Extensive use of POCUS in the setting of acute abdominal problems can potentially save significant healthcare resources (from both an organizational and economical point of view)
- *Investment in training* would be cost-worthy and rapidly amortized

Appendix: Chapter 11—Test Yourself (Answers in the Appendix at the End of the Book)

Q1—Routine use of SP-POCUS contribute to save and reduce:

- Time-to-decision-making.
- Money.
- Length of hospital stay.
- All of the above.

Further Reading

Barchiesi M, Bulgheroni M, Federici C, Casella F, Medico MD, Torzillo D, et al. Impact of point of care ultrasound on the number of diagnostic examinations in elderly patients admitted to an internal medicine ward. Eur J Intern Med. 2020;79:88–92. https://doi.org/10.1016/j.ejim.2020.06.026.

Bierig SM, Jones A. Accuracy and cost comparison of ultrasound versus alternative imaging modalities including CT, MR, PET, and angiography. J Diagn Med Sonogr. 2009;25(3):138–44. https://doi.org/10.1177/8756479309336240.

Bozzo S, Carrara G, Coppola S, Pirovano R, Zago M. Daily use of surgeon-performed ultrasound in a general and emergency surgery unit. Overall analysis of a two years prospective registry. *In* Abstracts. Eur J Trauma Emerg Surg. 2019;45(Suppl 1):1–264. https://doi.org/10.1007/s00068-019-01109-1.

Brogi E, Bignami E, Sidoti A, Shawar M, Gargani L, Vetrugno L, et al. Could the use of bedside lung ultrasound reduce the number of chest x-rays in the intensive care unit? Cardiovasc Ultrasound. 2017;15(1):23. https://doi.org/10.1186/s12947-017-0113-8.

D'Souza N, Marsden M, Bottomley S, Nagarajah N, Scutt F, Toh S. Cost-effectiveness of routine imaging of suspected appendicitis. Ann R Coll Surg Engl. 2018;100(1):47–51. https://doi.org/10.1308/rcsann.2017.0132.

Kurihara H, Zago M, Mariani D, Casamassima A, Luzzana F, Turconi MG, et al. Surgeon performed ultrasound for acute appendicitis. Can we decrease the number of negative appendectomies and avoid related economic loss? *In* Abstracts. Eur J Trauma. 2010;36(Suppl 1):1–238. https://doi.org/10.1007/s00068-010-8888-z.

Ministero della Salute, Repubblica Italiana. Rapporto annuale sull'attività di ricovero ospedaliero (Dati SDO 2018). http://www.salute.gov.it/imgs/C_17_pubblicazioni_2898_allegato.pdf.

Parker L, Nazarian LN, Carrino JA, Morrison WB, Grimaldi G, Frangos AJ, et al. Musculoskeletal imaging: medicare use, costs, and potential for cost substitution. J Am Coll Radiol. 2008;5(3):182–8. https://doi.org/10.1016/j.jacr.2007.07.016.

Pezzotta G, Masiero G, Malagnino A, Bozzo S, Brescacin A, Carrara G, Zago M. Cost and benefit analysis of surgeon-performed point-of-care ultrasound (SP-POCUS) supporting decision making in a General Surgery Department. MECOSAN 2023;124.

Shen G, Wang J, Fei F, Mao M, Mei Z. Bedside ultrasonography for acute appendicitis: an updated diagnostic meta-analysis. Int J Surg. 2019;70:1–9. https://doi.org/10.1016/j.ijsu.2019.08.009.

Soldati G, Testa A, Silva FR, Carbone L, Portale G, Silveri NG. Chest ultrasonography in lung contusion. Chest. 2006;130(2):533–8. https://doi.org/10.1378/chest.130.2.533.

Zago M, Mariani D, Casamassima A, Turconi MG, Kurihara H, Luzzana F. Chest X-ray can be safely skipped if thoracic US (EFAST) is included in trauma protocol – a prospective study. Eur J Trauma. 2008;34(Suppl 1):1–143. https://doi.org/10.1007/s00068-008-8001-4.

Chapter 13
Appendix: Test Yourself—Answers

Mauro Zago, Diego Mariani, and Marina Troian

Chapter 2

Q1—In the vast majority of cases, how many layers of a hollow viscus can you detect by US?

A1—3.

Comment: Even if there are five intestinal layers, trans-abdominal US allows you to see mainly three layers. Remember to use a linear probe for higher quality definition!

Q2—Normal peristalsis is easily detectable in the…

A2—Small bowel.

Comment: The appendix has no peristalsis; large bowel peristalsis is rarely detected by US.

Chapter 4

Q1—Look at Fig. 4.4. How dilated is the bowel loop?

A1—30 mm.

Comment: Have a look on the right side of the picture. There is a graded scale, each step corresponding to 10 mm. Remember that measuring the loop diameter is essential, as you can get an idea "at a glance."

Q2—What do you need to search for confirming an SBO on US?

A2—Empty distal small bowel.

M. Zago (✉)
General and Emergency Surgery Unit, General Surgery Department, ASST Lecco, "A. Manzoni" Hospital, Lecco, Italy

D. Mariani
Department of General Surgery, ASST Ovest Milanese, "Ospedale Nuovo" di Legnano, Legnano (Milan), Italy

M. Troian
Cardiothoracic and Vascular Department, ASUGI Cattinara University Hospital, Trieste, Italy

M. Zago et al. (eds.), *Point-of-care US for Acute Abdomen*,
https://doi.org/10.1007/978-3-031-40231-9_13

Comment: The detection of both empty distal ileum and dilated proximal small bowel loops is the easiest way to confirm SBO.

Chapter 5

Q1—A colonic diverticulum usually appears as…

A1—A hyperechoic round-shaped image surrounded by hypoechoic pericolic fat.

Comment: If in doubt, look again at Fig. 4.3, Chap. 4.

Q2—POCUS landmarks for finding the left colon are…?

A2—ASIS, iliac muscle, descending/sigmoid colon.

Comment: If it is still not clear, go back to Fig. 4.1, Chap. 4.

Chapter 6

Q1—The maximum normal diameter of the appendix is…?

A1—6 mm.

Comment: The bladder should preferably be empty when performing US for acute appendicitis.

Q2—POCUS landmarks for acute appendicitis are…?

A2—Cecum, psoas, iliac vessels, distal ileum.

Chapter 8

Q1—For getting the *Zenith sign*, you need to ask the patient to…

A1—Turn on the left side.

Q2—The peritoneal stripe thickening sign means…

A2—Bubbles of free air "trapped" behind the parietal peritoneum.

Chapter 9

Q1—Pre-stenotic dilation in Crohn's disease is defined as…?

A1—>25–30 mm.

Q2—Pathological thickening of a bowel wall is…

A2–>3 mm.

Chapter 10

Q1—CEUS is possible…

A1—If you have the software on the US equipment.

Comment: If in doubt, read again the "Scanning technique" paragraph in Chap. 9.

Chapter 11

Q1—Do you think E-FAST views can be useful for a right decision in a wide range of situations out of trauma settings?

Comment: This is a question challenging your mindset. If your answer is yes, we are pleased to share this knowledge with you. If your answer is no, we regret your decision and we hope you will be able to possibly change your mind in the future.

Chapter 12

Q1—Routine use of SP-POCUS contribute to save and reduce.

A1—All of the above.

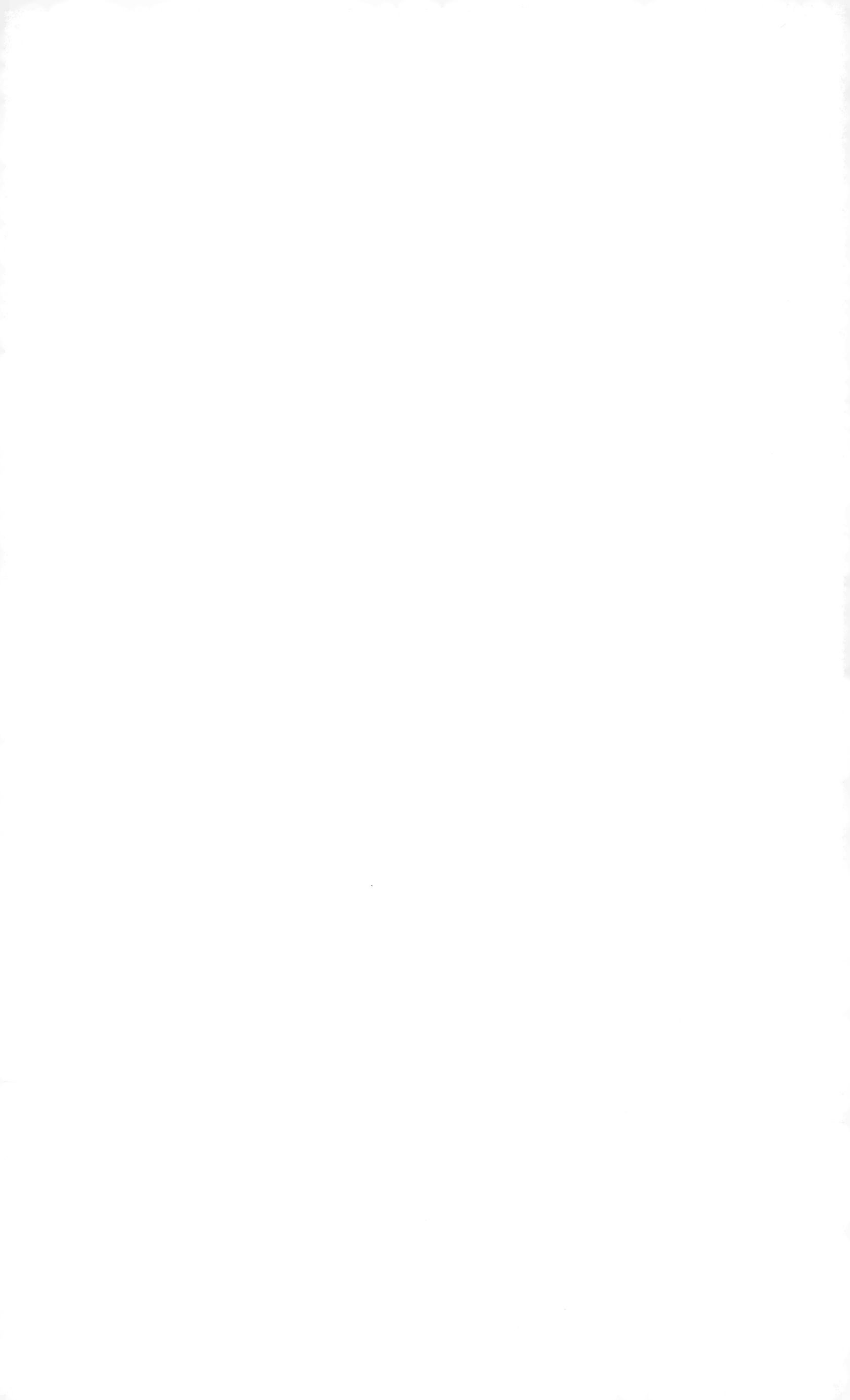

GPSR Compliance

The European Union's (EU) General Product Safety Regulation (GPSR) is a set of rules that requires consumer products to be safe and our obligations to ensure this.

If you have any concerns about our products, you can contact us on ProductSafety@springernature.com

In case Publisher is established outside the EU, the EU authorized representative is:

Springer Nature Customer Service Center GmbH
Europaplatz 3
69115 Heidelberg, Germany

Batch number: 10370712

Printed by Printforce, the Netherlands